D0595455

"I was really nervous about this book, but every family has its secrets. So what? Doesn't every mother pack a suitcase full of brisket to bring to her children? This book is about life and relationships and what happens when things don't go as planned. I guess all those years I dropped Aileen off at the library so I could get an hour to myself once in a while really paid off. This is a good story. You should read it. But I'm still leaving the country for a few weeks when it comes out."

—Mrs. Weintraub, Aileen's mom

Knocked Down

| AMERICAN LIVES | *Series editor:* Tobias Wolff |

Knocked Down

A High-Risk Memoir

Aileen Weintraub

University of Nebraska Press | *Lincoln*

The University of Nebraska Press is part of a land-grant institution with campuses and programs on the past, present, and future homelands of the Pawnee, Ponca, Otoe-Missouria, Omaha, Dakota, Lakota, Kaw, Cheyenne, and Arapaho Peoples, as well as those of the relocated Ho-Chunk, Sac and Fox, and Iowa Peoples.

Library of Congress Cataloging-in-Publication Data
Names: Weintraub, Aileen, 1973– author.
Title: Knocked down: a high-risk memoir / Aileen Weintraub.
Description: Lincoln: University of Nebraska Press, [2022] | Series: American lives
Identifiers: LCCN 2021036588
ISBN 9781496230201 (paperback)
ISBN 9781496231895 (epub)
ISBN 9781496231901 (pdf)
Subjects: LCSH: Weintraub, Aileen, 1973– | Pregnant women—Biography. | Bed rest. | Farm life. | BISAC: BIOGRAPHY & AUTOBIOGRAPHY / Personal Memoirs | BIOGRAPHY & AUTOBIOGRAPHY / Women
Classification: LCC HQ759 .W429 2022 | DDC 306.874/3—dc23
LC record available at https://lccn.loc.gov/2021036588

Set in ITC New Baskerville by Laura Buis.

To my father

Contents

Author's Note

This is a true story, even the parts where you will undoubtedly shake your head and say, "No way, did that really happen?" Some names and identifying features have been changed to mildly protect the identity of certain individuals. Minor tweaks to the timeline of events were made for literary cohesion.

Knocked Down

1 | Roots Run Deep

The house was haunted.

I had my suspicions when I moved in. In the middle of the night, the lights flickered, the phone chimed when nobody called, and most disturbing, I witnessed tears sliding down the rough, misshapen stone fireplace. Maybe it was because my father-in-law's ashes were kept in a German beer stein on the mantel. Or because one day my husband's grandmother put her head down on the dining room table as though she were about to take a nap and died instead.

The child inside my belly would be the fourth generation to live here. Unfortunately, it had also been four generations since anyone had slapped a coat of paint on the walls or updated the furniture. But I loved the place, an old dairy farm my husband, Chris, had inherited, and we planned to spend the rest of our lives fixing it up and making it our own.

I surveyed the room, the dusty old Victrola that played by itself, the pastel vertical blinds that rattled when there was no breeze. I was going to start crying just like my fireplace if I had to look at all this for one more day. Perhaps a little sprucing up would act as a peace offering to the spirits for invading their space. I needed to stay occupied, otherwise I would succumb to a loop of anxiety. I was twenty weeks pregnant and had been on bed rest for fourteen days, getting up only to pee and to take a quick shower. That meant I had twenty weeks to go in my sentence of near-solitary confinement . . . if I was lucky enough to make it to my due date. My only crime: an ailing cervix.

Two weeks earlier I had been spread-eagle on the examination table in a bright yellow room looking up at a poster of an imitation Georgia O'Keeffe flower taped to the ceiling while my doctor put her hands in places that generally required a lot more foreplay and at least a little bit of booze. Fashionably decked out in one of those fabulous pink paper robes, which had ripped as I slipped it on, I looked like I was sporting some cheap off-the-shoulder evening wear. It was the first time my husband had seen me in stirrups. So much for maintaining *that* air of mystery, but his eyes twinkled when he looked at me, and I was reassured.

I propped myself up on my elbows to get a better look at the doctor, who was mumbling something between my legs, but all I could see were the dark roots on her bleached-blond head. I lay back down and gave Chris a smile and a wink. He was doing well, sitting off to my right in the unofficial husband's chair. We had planned to go to that little Mexican place down on the waterfront for dinner, and I began thinking about the menu options.

Then the doctor made her pronouncement, and my life changed.

"Wait, what?" I heard Chris say.

In an instant, my eyes had fixed on my husband's darkened demeanor. In place of the reassurance I had seen moments earlier, there was fear. *No, no*, I thought, shaking my head. The doctor's shiny red lips moved, but I absorbed just bits: ". . . cervix . . . situation . . . dangerous."

Now here I was in bed, a commitment-phobic Brooklyn girl stuck in a haunted farmhouse for the next five months with my husband gone most of the day, and no one around to hear me scream. So that's what I did. I threw my head back on the pillow and let out a bloodcurdling howl of rage and fear and sadness that reverberated down to the deepest part of my core and filled the room, bouncing off the old windowpanes.

The house shook. I looked around as if challenging even the spirits to answer me but was met only with deafening silence. Then I rolled onto my side and fixed my gaze at the sun setting over the horizon, turning the sky a brilliant orange, streaked with reds, golds, and the softest pinks. I stayed like that until dark, a thick round tear sliding across the bridge of my nose, splashing onto the comforter.

There was only one person who could get me through this. But he wasn't here. And I needed him now more than ever.

2 | A GORE-TEX Primer

Five Years before Bed Rest

"Are you out of your fuckin' mind?" my father asked as he reached over to pour a cup of coffee for me from the old-fashioned percolator.

I had just told my parents over Entenmann's crumb cake that I planned to quit my job at a children's publishing company in Manhattan. I yearned for windows with a view and air that had not been recycled through ventilation systems.

"For once in your life would ya just stick with something?" My father banged his fist on the table for emphasis, though not particularly hard.

I traced my fingers along one of the pink and blue flowers on the kitchen wallpaper in the house where I had grown up. "I haven't found anything I like just yet." I shrugged.

"You quit everything."

"I do not quit everything. I just try a lot more things than most people."

My mother stood up from the table. "Is this going to be like the time you quit Brownies? Robin Schumaker's mother said there was no more room, but she finally agreed to squeeze you in. And then you quit." She pulled out a chair, climbed up, and began rearranging glassware on the top shelf of the cabinet.

"I was five! They made me dunk for apples. All those little mouths reaching into that big bowl like piranhas."

"How about Arizona?"

"Let's just make a list," I said.

Some people pick a college based on academics or sports programs. I looked at a map and picked the farthest possible point from my parents' house. My college experience in Arizona lasted all of five minutes before I did an about-face back to the East Coast. My dormmates had never met a Jewish girl before, and when I referred to pizza as a pie, they had no idea what I was talking about. I knew I'd never fit in.

"Do you ever think about getting married?" my mother asked, looming over me on the chair.

I looked up at her. "How could I not when you've been asking me that question since I was four years old?" I reached to grab a Macy's catalog from a pile of mail on the flaking yellow radiator and began flipping through.

"Nice Jewish girls go to college, get married, and have babies. Tell her, Richard."

"It's true," my father said, nodding.

Getting married and becoming a mother was my fate. It had been drilled into my head since I was a preschooler and my mother made me practice swaddling my Holly Hobby doll. Now here I was at twenty-six listening to how I had failed to live up to my parents' grand plans.

"Do you want me to find you someone?" my mother asked as she turned back to the cabinet. Perhaps she'd find someone up there.

"No, I don't want you to find me someone." I folded down a page of the catalog, noting a pair of Steve Madden boots.

My father shook his head, taking a sip of coffee. "Boy, do I feel sorry for *him*," he murmured into his cup. As if this "him" was just waiting in the wings to take over my parents' burden of dealing with me. This hypothetical man I was to marry and procreate with had been talked up and personified so much it began to feel like a *Where's Waldo?* game. I just had to find him among a plethora of funny-looking characters and striped shirts.

"This quitting your job nonsense—bad idea, Kabeen," my father continued, and I could tell the lecture was almost over. He had been calling me Kabeen all my life, and when he said it now, I knew he was resigned. My father worried that whatever decisions I made would either kill me or, worse, mean I'd have to move back into their house.

"Hebrew school!" my mother shouted out as though she had just solved the final puzzle on *Wheel of Fortune*. She turned to face me, nodding triumphantly, still on the chair and holding the Shabbat candlesticks she was preparing for Friday night's dinner.

"Yes, Mom. I'm a Hebrew school dropout. I will carry that shame for the rest of my life."

My father leaned in. "I was actually proud of you for that one," he whispered. "Saved me on the bat mitzvah." He winked at me. We were observant Jews at my mother's insistence, but my father only begrudgingly went along.

"I dropped out of Hebrew school because Mark used to beat the daylights out of me on the walk home."

"I really wish you and your brother got along." My mother sighed.

She hopped off the chair, set the Shabbat candles on the stove top, and began scooping out the melted wax from the previous week with a butter knife.

"Think this through, Kabeen," my father warned, taking the last forkful of crumb cake.

So that's what I did.

While trying to sort out this latest dilemma, I booked a trip to Alaska to clear my head. While there, I strapped on crampons for the first time and climbed a glacier. On that massive chunk of ice, two older Canadian men with thick beards, whom I had just met moments before, offered to suspend me over a deep, plummeting crevasse so I could peer into oblivion. Each took one of my arms, and with total trust, I leaned all the way forward. The frigid wind whipped my hair around, the cold stinging my eyes. I could see the hard, unforgiving ice and the blue water rushing beneath. I could see both the permanent and the temporary, the sharp edges, the sacredness of it all. The very second I was upright I knew that I would never work in an office again. I had looked into the depths of eternity, and there were no cubicles down there.

I had never considered leaving the city, but now I could see the grandness of nature, which I was clearly missing, surrounded instead by lunch trucks, orange and white steam pipes, and relentless jackhammers. After Alaska I began looking for a way out of my comfort zone and back into the sense of reverence I had felt on that glacier. Perhaps there was a life for me beyond the city.

I signed up for an outdoor educational program through AmeriCorps (what I thought of as Peace Corps lite) that would take me to the wilderness of upstate New York. I would be educating children, building trails, and doing completely unglamorous things like shoveling piles of rocks out of trailers. My father was livid. He couldn't believe I was quitting my job "to live in the woods with the freaks," as he put it. He stopped talking to me and refused to help me move out of my Victorian Bay Ridge apartment, a rare find. Affordable, an open floor plan, original sconces—I knew I'd never rent another one like it. After handing the keys over to my landlord, I spent the night celebrating my twenty-seventh birthday dancing on the bar at the famous Hogs and Heifers Saloon in the Meatpacking District, my girlfriends and I tossing our bras into the crowd. I stayed at my parents' house for the next three days before heading into the woods. Each time I passed my father in the long hallway, he gave me a sidelong look of exasperation, mumbling under his breath. His disappointment broke my heart.

On the first day of the AmeriCorps program, I showed up to the trailhead in a pair of bright red Urban Outfitters corduroys and hiking boots with two-inch platform heels.

"Weintraub, you're going to need to be waterproof. Get yourself some GORE-TEX," snapped the corps leader, a rugged thirtysomething backwoods boy.

"What's GORE-TEX?" I whispered to the girl standing next to me. She gave me the once-over and then lifted the collar of her jacket as if that were supposed to clear the whole thing up. The next morning I overheard a discussion about frost warnings and black ice; the former sounded ominous, while I assumed the latter was just country-speak for dirty snow. I was definitely outside my comfort zone.

By the end of that week, I started to get with the program, rising at dawn for early morning hikes, donning thermals and trail runners, and tying back my unruly blond curls into a sensible ponytail. By the third week I was slamming my very own pickax against concrete to refurbish a Habitat for Humanity house. The corps leader walked by and whispered in my ear, "You surprised me. Figured you would have flagged down the first Greyhound and hightailed it out of here by now."

I went home for Rosh Hashanah wondering if my father was talking to me yet. He refused to go to synagogue, so we went without him. While my mother, brother, and I were Conservative Jews, he had been raised Reformed and didn't feel a spiritual pull to sit in temple for three hours listening to prayers in a language he didn't understand. This stratification of Judaism is confusing, so I'll explain it as it relates to bacon. In Judaism the major players are: Reformed—eat bacon and love it; Conservative—eat bacon only in diners; Orthodox— never touch bacon but secretly wonder what it tastes like; Ultra-Orthodox—no way, feh, it's *treif*; and Chassidic—what is this bacon of which you speak?

On a few occasions my mother had caught my father practicing his own special version of Judaism in the house, like cooking steak in a frying pan instead of in the broiler. (According to Jewish law, meat cannot be cooked in a pan unless it has been soaked and salted to make sure the blood has first been drained.) If my mother unexpectedly came home while my father was cooking steak this way, he'd yell to me and my brother in code, "We've got to paint the house," and we'd all scramble to hide the evidence, opening windows and spraying Lysol to get rid of the fumes. My mother was never fooled.

After returning from morning prayer, I sat down on the floor next to him while he watched football, or maybe it was hockey.

"You like it up there?" His cigarette burned a thin thread through the air.

"It's okay." And that was it.

My father was my best friend, and it weighed on me when we disagreed. I was relieved we were past this latest quarrel. That evening, after stuffing ourselves with egg salad, *kneidlach*, *tzimmes*, and other holiday fare, I sat on his lap in his Archie Bunker chair while we gathered in the living room. He was soft and rounding with age, and when I placed my head on his shoulder, I could feel his flesh give.

The next morning, before I left to go back upstate to my AmeriCorps post, I went into my parents' bedroom to say goodbye. My mother had left for work, but my father was still sleeping. He always slept on his side with one hand resting under his stubbled cheek. He had a partial grin as though his dreams were lovely. I kissed him on his brow and then gently patted down his too-long, brownish-gray hair, which he always insisted was blond.

A little over a week later, I received a voice mail from my mother that my father needed emergency stomach surgery. No biggie. The stomach isn't near any major organs. I'd talk to him in the morning. Still, I sat vigil by the phone waiting for word that he was okay. At midnight my mother called again. Everything was fine, she said, but I could sense a commotion in the background. She quickly hung up. I felt sick. A deep instinct pushed me homeward. I gathered a few corps members to give me a ride back to the city, a four-hour drive in the middle of the night. Cell service didn't yet exist in that part of upstate New York so I had no way to get updates.

When I arrived my brother opened the door to my family's two-story brick house. Standing on the red stoop, the same stoop where my father had taught me to button up my crimson faux-fur coat that he had designed himself while working in the garment industry, the same red stoop where he had shown me how to hit a baseball with my plastic bat and years later snuck me my first drag of a cigarette, that was the place where my brother looked at me and sobbed, "He's dead." Somehow I had already known.

My father had been on blood thinners, and they "just couldn't get the blood to clot." An aneurysm, the doctor had said. The surgeon told my mother that he kept pouring and pouring blood into my father, but nothing worked. I didn't know exactly what he meant by "pouring," but I envisioned him standing over my father's open body with measuring cups. My mother invited the corps members who'd driven me home into the house to eat, but I knew better and asked them to give us privacy. I shut the door, climbed up the long flight of steps to our house, and pressed my wet face to the hallway wall to keep from collapsing on the floor, where my mother and brother were wailing in each other's arms. "I wasn't finished. We weren't finished," I cried over and over, slamming my hand into the wall. We had so much more to talk about; I had so much more to learn from him.

It is tradition that Jews bury their own dead. Most of the time, it's through a symbolic gesture in which each mourner takes a turn shoveling a small amount of dirt over the casket. Whatever is left, the gravediggers complete. "It means we take care of our own," my mother told us. I was in the front row during the graveside service, and when I turned to take the shovel, I saw that over a hundred people had shown up, no small surprise since my father was a pretty solitary guy who hated just about everyone he met.

I threw a pile of dirt on my father's coffin and put the shovel in the ground for the next person. And then I noticed, after each person had taken a turn, instead of going back to their cars, they stayed. They kept shoveling. I looked around at the faces of the friends I had grown up with, their parents, and cousins I hadn't seen in years. We would do the job ourselves.

I climbed to the top of the big dirt mound and began shoveling heavy loads of earth, rain pouring down, streaks of mud not only on my face but on the faces of all the mourners. This was what it meant to have community. More shovels appeared, perhaps from the gravediggers standing discreetly off to the side. The hole was almost filled, the wet ground devouring the simple maple coffin, when my mother's shriek pierced the quick cadence of dirt being heaped into the grave. "Wait! I can't find my keys!" she yelled. We all stopped and looked at her, then toward the grave. She rifled through her purse. "They may have fallen in!" I looked down at my clothing, my red shirt stained brown. My father's good friend Paulie, his suit ruined and his yarmulke sliding off his head, stood next to his grown sons, and all were poised to either start digging or continue shoveling. "Okay, okay," my mother called out, "I found them. Thank God, we don't have to dig him up. Keep going."

Her friend Zahava came up beside her. "Gail, we'll get through this together." And then she wrapped my mother in her arms.

After the funeral, we sat Shiva for a week. I couldn't relate to the ritual of sitting on wooden boxes while people streamed through our home offering us chunks of babka and other cakes, paying awkward condolences. By the third day, my best friend from childhood, Rachel, an Orthodox Jew who had married right out of college and already had two kids, told me to take a break and come over to her house, where she handed me a big bowl of ice cream and led me to her couch. "Cry. That's what you need to do. I'm going shopping for Shabbat." After she left with her kids in tow, I put the bowl with the already melting ice cream on the end table and stared at a small crack in the wall for the next two hours.

I stayed in AmeriCorps for another two and a half months, try- ing to pretend it was no big deal, his death. But I cried every night, and familiar Brooklyn was calling me home. I packed my duffle, wondering if my father would be disappointed in me for quitting. Or would he understand this time? I moved in with my mother, who was now alone in a big house, and began focusing on my freelance-writing career.

Then two months after my twenty-eighth birthday, a little over a year after my father died, I headed back to the country, this time taking both my North Face GORE-TEX and my Tahari evening wear, feeling that I had some unfinished business left "in the woods with the freaks." I wanted to be outdoors again, to hike, to gaze upon fall colors and expansive views. Alaska had crystalized that for me. I was born in Brooklyn. I came from Brooklyn, but that borough's deep vibration of elevated subway cars and flashing neon signs no longer felt right. This time I wouldn't be heading back to the camarade- rie of AmeriCorps. Now I would find my own way.

As I was packing the last of my belongings, standing in my childhood bedroom, I began to understand why my father had been so against my leaving Brooklyn. He didn't want me to go. It was as simple as that. It wasn't because he was afraid I'd never make enough money to support myself or that I'd be eaten by bears; it was that he wanted me to stay close to home.

I don't know that it would have stopped me, this knowledge, but it would have made me understand how deeply he loved me. I stood there for a moment longer, forgetting the task at hand. There is a saying that a boy becomes a man when he loses his father. But what about a girl? What does she become?

3 | Produce Man

Three Years before Bed Rest

Saugerties, a sleepy Hudson Valley town with big shop windows, narrow streets, and an old-fashioned movie theater, surrounded by large tracts of farmland, was known as "the place time forgot." Two hours north of New York City, it was too far for commuters, so it felt like a world away. This was where I planned to grieve, heal, and write. I rented a garden apartment in this small, obscure town, basing my choice solely on the fact that the landlord was a jazz musician who referred to himself in third person as "Sattan from Manhattan."

In an attempt to make a living, I conjured up an extravagant plan that would rocket-launch my writing career and catapult me into fame and stardom. I had already had a few children's books published, but now I was going to focus on a new humorous memoir about dating. Lord knows I had enough experience. I had spent years primping, plotting, and, yes, even praying, driven toward the one unequivocal goal of marrying and procreating. The thought of being an "old" bride was more than I could bear.

I began attending Friday night services at the local synagogue in hopes of meeting *the one* but had instead stumbled upon the geriatric faction of upstate Jews. An older woman in a sleeveless dress plastered with orange begonias jutted her chin at my modest cleavage and said, "Why would a young girl come to temple alone on a Friday night?" In other words, I wasn't welcome. I had to accept that the pickings in this tiny town were slim. As for searching for my soul mate online, it was early 2002 and internet dating was just becoming a thing, especially in upstate New York, so it wasn't on my radar.

My family and community had pressured me into getting married for so long, I wasn't even sure if I was doing this for them or for myself. All I knew was I had put so much thought into seducing my future husband and father of my child that I had enough material to write a book titled *The Ten-Second Seduction*. The premise was that when you meet a man, you know within ten seconds whether or not you feel that electrifying zing—the one that says you must absolutely see that person again . . . naked. Ten seconds doesn't sound like a lot, but I was efficient. Every chapter would be named after a single identifying characteristic of a man I had dated. There was, for example, Mr. Spirituality, who thought sex could only happen on a higher spiritual plane. (I didn't have that kind of time to learn to levitate.) Then of course there was Dr. Broccoli, who had an unnatural fear of the vegetable, Motorcycle Man, Military Man, Green Underwear Guy . . . The list was long. My plan was to transform myself into *the* comic seduction expert of Ulster County.

Every writer has their props. Sometimes it's a much-loved teacup or books about writing, a special pen, or a poster with a meaningful quote. Mine was a faux diamond–studded tiara. I'd whip that baby out of its box, place it on my head, and begin crafting my prose.

Overall, things were going well, and after a year of adjusting to life in a small town, though I was barely making it from one paycheck to the next from freelance-writing gigs, I was building a life for myself. The best part? There was not a cubicle in sight.

I would like to say that I was so engaged with my writing I forgot to eat for days at a time, but the truth was, I had a bad habit of spending the little money I had on books and shoes rather than on decent food. It had gotten to a point where

I was eating Cheerios sandwiches on white bread with Russian dressing for breakfast. One morning, as I sat in front of my computer, I stopped and looked at my sandwich, Russian dressing dripping down the side of my wrist. A half hour later I was standing over a row of fruit in the produce section of the grocery store when a tall, muscular man wearing a baseball cap appeared to my right.

"You don't want those grapes," he said, picking out his own.

"No?" I was intrigued. Out of the corner of my eye, I noticed the curve of his bicep and his long limbs. I stood up straighter and hoped to God I didn't have Russian dressing stains on my sweater.

"They're rotten. You can tell by the dried-up stems."

I scanned the vegetable section to make sure this man didn't have a wife standing over by the asparagus, and then I tilted my head toward him. Our eyes connected for a split second. I smiled. And then he pushed his cart off in the direction of the dairy aisle. My gaze fell on his broad shoulders and his blue T-shirt clinging to his delicious trapezius muscles. It took restraint, but I did *not* run up behind him, jump on his back, wrap my arms around his chest, and bite the flesh just below his neck.

It was complete infatuation at first sight; clearly the man had just saved me from consuming bad fruit and dying from some, well, bad fruit disease. I owed him everything. I know. The produce section. How cliché. This was *so* going in *The Ten-Second Seduction*: Produce Man.

As fate would have it, I met up with him once again in the tomato sauce aisle. This time I was prepared.

"Arrabiata or Alfredo?" I asked.

"Depends what you're making. Don't spend too much, but don't sacrifice quality." He reached over and grabbed a jar of sauce to examine the ingredients.

I nearly swooned.

We discussed the merits of pasta sauce until the conversation turned personal. He lived in the Bronx but was upstate visiting his ailing father, which explained the older man with a bandage around his head circling the aisle with a shopping cart. The third time his father came around, grazing his cart into Produce Man's heels, he told me he was sorry but he had to go, and he asked for my contact information.

We emailed back and forth for about two weeks—this was before texting—and I learned that Produce Man worked for a hedge fund in New York City but often came upstate on the weekends to stay with his father. When I mentioned I had just purchased new hiking boots, he asked if I'd like to join him for a day in the Catskill Mountains. I wasn't sure I wanted to head into the woods with a complete stranger, so I suggested we meet in a public place—the mall. I hadn't met a boy at the mall since I was sixteen.

My very first date with Produce Man landed on the second anniversary of my father's death. I took this as a sign that my father had sent him from the heavens and it was *bashert*, the Jewish term for "destiny."

We had planned dinner and a movie. No grand gestures here, but I was surprisingly content with this. We never made it to the movie, instead talking well into the evening. He was soft-spoken and refined and looked no older than twenty-five, even though he was in his thirties. He told me that after college he had lived in Brazil, competing professionally as a jiu-jitsu fighter, and then went back to school years later to get a master's of science with a focus in chemistry from Columbia University. He wasn't Jewish, but he lived with someone who was—a wealthy elderly woman in Riverdale who had rented him a room in her mansion in exchange for errands and the security of having another human being in the house.

"You keep kosher?" I asked when he told me they often ate meals together.

"Rent in the city is pretty steep. Small price to pay."

"And being kosher is no problem for you?"

"Nope." He was a man of few words, but that was okay because I had so much to say.

"I've never met a kosher Christian before."

"You have now."

By the end of the evening, this beautiful man was sitting in front of me practically reciting the laws of kashrus. Not only that, he was already used to taking care of a little old Jewish lady. One day I would be a little old Jewish lady!

Sitting in his own car as he watched me settle into mine, he leaned out the window resting his chin on crossed arms, smiling at me with his boyish grin. I drove away thinking, *Quiet, maybe, but I bet I could make him talk.*

By our third date, though he swears it was our second, I had invited him into my apartment. Within moments we were sliding across the length of the kitchen counter, knocking over cups, unaware of the paper towel roll unraveling across the floor, my legs wrapped around his strong body as he hoisted me up to eye level. I playfully bit his lip. This guy was reserved, but I could see a passion simmering beneath the surface.

"Would you like a drink?" I said, and then shimmied out from under him, hiding my flushed face in the refrigerator as I pretended to rummage around for a beer.

That was when I began referring to Produce Man by his real name, Chris. I even allowed myself to entertain the slightest possibility that perhaps my book *The Ten-Second Seduction* would culminate in one resounding, triumphant chapter where I had found "him" at last.

And so I had.

4 | Cricket Hill

Two Years before Bed Rest

Spring arrived and we planted a huge garden in the backyard of Chris's family home in Accord, New York, a forty-minute drive from Saugerties. His father had succumbed to leukemia, and Chris had inherited the old dairy farm nestled in the woods. When Chris was young, his parents divorced, so he had never lived on the farm, but since it had been in his family for generations, he had spent many weekends and holidays there. Now he was brimming with plans to make it his own.

The house was sturdy but needed TLC. We began by building a garden fence—that is, I told Chris where I thought the posts should go and picked out the size of the chicken wire. Then I went to the local hardware store and bought seeds based on the colors of the packaging.

"How do these work?" I said mostly to myself, ripping open a packet. Chris was busy digging out a stubborn root.

"Horseradish," he said, holding up his victory prize.

"Horseradish is red. *That* would not be on my Seder plate."

"Add beets." He tossed the muddy, twisted root at me. I stepped back, watching it land at my feet.

"I'm not touching that." I nudged the top of it with my foot.

Chris bent over and picked it up. "Good stuff." He dangled it in front of me, the piquant odor driving into my nostrils. This was a root vegetable on steroids.

Chris went back to digging and I went back to breathing and reading my seed packets. I refused to admit my lack of expertise when it came to planting seeds, so I began just sprinkling them all over the place, hoping he didn't notice.

The more delicate ones didn't make it, but weeks later, when I finally saw the fruits of our labor in the tiny budding sprouts of kale and radish, I knew our relationship had catapulted to the next level. If you plant a garden with someone, you are basically saying to that person that you plan to be around to share the bounty. *Seduction.*

Chris was still spending weekdays in the city, and I loved that I could visit him there. We went to Broadway shows together and strolled around SoHo. He took me on shopping sprees along Fifth Avenue, buying me purses and books, and we checked out hot new restaurants. At the end of each date, before jumping on the subway, we'd find a park bench in Union Square and people-watch.

I'd never dated a man who could work a chain saw and ride a tractor, all while explaining quantum mechanics. He dropped money like he had plenty of it, but wasn't wasteful, and he was introducing me to haute cuisine, which was vastly different from Cheerios sandwiches with Russian dressing. He was sexy and exotic. I knew he must have flaws, but I didn't want to see them just yet.

Back on the farm, aptly named Cricket Hill, we'd sit outside on rickety metal rocking chairs late at night, gazing at the stars. With the cacophonous chirping of crickets and cicadas, the howling coyotes and hooting owls, I thought it odd that the country was considered a place for quiet contemplation.

"So, what is it you like about me, anyway?" I asked one night.

He paused a moment. "You talk a lot."

"People don't usually consider that a good quality." *What about my blue eyes, my sparkling wit?*

"I don't know. I'm pretty quiet. It's good to have someone fill the silence."

"Anything else?" *My golden hair? My thirst for knowledge? My ass?*

"You're a spitfire. You moved up here all by yourself without knowing anyone. That's pretty brave."

Nobody had ever complimented me for speaking my mind and being courageous. This was big. I wondered if he would always feel this way.

Cricket Hill was made up of acres and acres of lush green land, and that night Chris promised to build me a castle, one with a tower, so I could lean out the window and call to him. It was fun, silly talk, but somehow, in the haze of this affair, I believed it. We talked about our future and how many children we were going to have. "Six for me," I said, and though I could see the look of shock flit across his face, he simply replied, "We'll talk about it."

Late Sunday evenings Chris escorted me to my car and we lingered in the driveway, kissing and chatting, before he headed back to the city and I returned to my little apartment in Saugerties. I drove home, head dizzy with lust, listening to our local radio host playing songs by Frank Sinatra. Chris and I shared a love of Sinatra—or, more accurately, our fathers had. My father's tombstone even bears the engraving, "He Did It His Way." We daydreamed that our dads would have gotten along splendidly watching Formula One racing, drinking whiskey, and talking politics.

Around this time, it was becoming more difficult to sustain myself on my writer's salary, and although I had almost finished the first draft of *The Ten-Second Seduction*, I was only just starting to contact agents and publishing houses. I also had a moral dilemma now. It was one thing for Chris to date a yet-to-be-revealed self-proclaimed comic seduction expert, but would he want the whole world to read about her previous exploits? Perhaps it was time for me to hang up my tiara. I would hold off sending out any more queries.

Though I longed for Chris during the week, and money was tight, the real problem was centipedes. They were taking over my apartment.

One morning, as Chris and I sat on my steps soaking in the unseasonably warm November sun, I mentioned I was thinking about going home to Brooklyn to find an office job. You know, because there are no vermin in Brooklyn.

"I need to make more money. I'm signing the lease over to the centipedes."

"Don't let the centipedes win."

"This isn't just about the centipedes. I'm done here. I mean, not with you. I like you. Just with this apartment."

It was half bluff, but we'd been dating for about a year, and it was time to make a move. Chris had this mostly empty house, and I was always there anyway. So after long discussions about arthropods and our future, we decided to both move into the farmhouse full time. Chris became animated as we planned the details; he hated the soulless hedge fund work. He would quit his job and look for employment upstate. Maybe he would invest in a small business, something he had always wanted to do. We spoke tentatively, excited about putting down roots. My father's voice echoed in my head: "Try not to screw this one up, would ya?"

My old '94 champagne Honda was packed to the hilt as I drove down the desolate country road that led to Cricket Hill. Like many New Yorkers raised on mass transit, I mistrusted my driving abilities. But it was with pride that I claimed this as my road, my home, my new life. It didn't matter that the house was dusty and old, that it was filled with generations of furniture and bric-a-brac. I loved the house for its character, for the future it represented, and I marveled at the view of the rocky blue Shawangunk Ridge.

Saugerties had been a booming metropolis compared to Accord. There, I could walk to a small grocery store and a coffee shop; here, the only thing within walking distance was the mailbox across the road. But on the afternoon I moved my belongings into the house, I stood on the deck overlooking the huge three-level field and saw endless possibilities for swing sets, swimming pools, farm animals, and boisterous family gatherings.

We quickly fell into a domestic routine, and on Sundays, after stacking wood, weeding, and beginning the long, arduous process of putting the gardens to bed in preparation for winter, we drove around the county looking for llama and alpaca owners to see if owning them was a feasible idea (there turned out to be only one, so we stalked him until he agreed to talk to us). I took this as a sign that a marriage proposal was imminent. It is a fact that if you are looking to raise llamas with another person, you are seriously considering a lifelong commitment to each other. These animals can live over twenty years. You do not want to battle in court over the custody of a llama.

When I mentioned what my weekends were like to my closest childhood friend, Rachel, she amped up her displeasure about my relationship.

"I don't like that you're living together," she said bluntly.

"It's okay. I'm hoping to get engaged soon," I said, thinking that was the issue.

"Oh," she said.

I had dated non-Jews ever since I was a teenager, and it had been a sore subject. Upon having my first kiss at fourteen, I ran home to call Rachel with the details, and though she was interested, she prefaced her inquiries with whether or not the boy was Jewish. But now we were talking high-stakes lifetime commitment.

"I really love this guy."

"You can really love a Jew just as easily. You have an obligation to marry within your religion."

This was true for Rachel, since as an Orthodox Jew, if you marry outside your religion, your community disowns you. I couldn't even pretend Christopher was Jewish. He had the word "Christ" in his name, for crying out loud. It's easy to say that Rachel had no right to tell me who to marry, that she and my other Orthodox friends weren't worth my time if they couldn't accept me for who I was and the choices I made. But Rachel had introduced me to the people in the Jewish organization Hillel, at Brooklyn College, where I eventually landed after the Arizona fiasco. Together we planned overnight Shabbat parties and dinners. We all practiced religious devotion at our own level. Some dressed modestly and vowed not to touch a boy until their wedding day; others wore jeans, held hands, and were more intimate with their future husbands. Though, unlike my secular friends, we never discussed the details of that intimacy.

My very first apartment was practically a sorority house for Orthodox girls. Some Friday evenings I spent at home with them, and on others I went clubbing in Manhattan until 8:00 a.m. I had straddled this line where I could either pursue a pious life or give it up altogether. I knew I'd never be Orthodox now, and I was figuring out how much I'd still practice, but marrying Chris would mean the certain end of invitations to big Shabbat dinners, and the love and security that came along with them.

"Aileen, if you marry him, I won't come to your wedding."

I had been a bridesmaid in Rachel's wedding, and though I figured she probably wouldn't be standing at my chuppah, it hadn't occurred to me that she wouldn't even show up. I knew that once Rachel threw down the gauntlet, many of my other Orthodox friends would follow suit.

I was in love and happy, but Rachel could not see the beauty in it. To her it was as if I had poisoned somebody or committed murder, but all I had done was open my heart. I was making a choice, and I chose love.

Fortunately, I had one friend who stood by me. If there were ever a male version of myself, Watson was it. We'd met years before in a creative writing class at Brooklyn College taught by a professor who was always drunk by 10:00 a.m. Watson's real name was Ed, but our teacher had a penchant for Sherlock Holmes references. I looked over at Ed one day and decided to change his name. We spent hours talking about writing, life, and of course how bad our professor was and, in the process, became lifelong friends. He was married now, two kids, nice house in the suburbs, but none of that had dulled his sharp-witted tongue.

So when I told Watson, who was also a Conservative Jew, about Rachel's reaction, he said, "This Chris person, do you love him?"

"Of course I love him."

"Every time you meet someone you tell me you're in love. What's so great about this one?"

"Well, he's . . . kind."

"He's kind? What bullshit is that?"

"No, really kind. And he fixes things. And he's smart, but humble. Plus, he said we could get a puppy. I've always wanted a puppy."

"I'm bored."

"But that's the thing! There's no drama. I'm sick of so much upheaval. I quit my job to become a freelancer, which is really stressful by the way, because apparently I like eating more than I thought; my father's dead; my mother and I drive each other bonkers. Chris offers me solace. He's funny, too. Other people can't read him, but I can. They ask me, 'What does Chris think?' Or, 'What does Chris want?' But no one will ask him because he's so quiet and also maybe because he can kill you with some fancy one-fingered jiu-jitsu. I like that. He shows this stoic side to the world and saves his heart for me. He provides me with peace and protects my solitude."

"Okay, I'm vomiting. But that's what I wanted you to hear yourself say."

"So, how do I give up Rachel and a whole community of people I really like?"

"Look, I don't know what your definition of a true friend is, but my friends want what's best for me, not what's best for them."

I knew Watson was onto something, but a part of me felt that pleasing Rachel also meant pleasing God, as if she were middle management.

So I did what any self-respecting Jewish girl would do when she is thinking of finally getting married. I called my mother.

"Will you keep kosher?" She had stumped me with the first question. I always assumed I'd keep a kosher home, but I had yet to discuss it with Chris.

"I guess that's a conversation Chris and I still need to have."

"Well, he's not Jewish, but what *is* he exactly?" She knew I was getting serious with Chris but had saved up her pressing questions until now in case he turned out not to be the one.

"Nonpracticing."

"What are his parents?"

"Don't know. His dad spoke Germ—I think his family were Austrian farmers."

"You're dating a German?"

"He's not German. He's Austrian."

"How do you know? They moved the borders every other day. One day you're Austrian, the next day you're calling yourself the Führer and killing an entire population. You couldn't date an Italian?"

"Because Mussolini was so nice to the Jews, Ma? The war is over. His family came here to escape the Nazis. He's never even been to Germany."

"Well, I'd like to meet him."

"So, does this mean you're okay with me marrying someone who's not Jewish?"

"Does this mean you're going to let me meet him?"

"Maybe I should get the ring first."

"Listen, of course I want you to marry a Jew," she said. "But more important, you should get married. And you should be happy. What would your father say?"

"Well, Chris has a lot of patience, and I'm pretty sure Dad would think that was a requirement to marry me." I believed that in some cosmic way he had chosen Chris.

"Would they get along?"

"I think so. As much as Dad got along with anybody." There was a big part of me that still wanted my father's approval. "Chris is well-read, like Dad, especially when it comes to history. He doesn't care about religion, much like Dad. And I think he would appreciate Dad's sense of humor."

"Will your kids be Jewish?" She'd given up on my salvation but figured she could try again with the next generation.

"It's not like I'm giving up Judaism."

"As long as your kids are Jewish and you love him, it'll be fine."

Between Watson and my mother, I had my answer. Now, if only Chris would ask the question.

A few months later, Chris and I were visiting the Saugerties Lighthouse when he sat down on a cornerstone and pulled me onto his lap. It was a cloudless August day, and together we gazed upon the horizon, listening to the sound of water crest gently over the shoreline. He turned me to face him, and I could feel his body tense and then relax. It's one of those moments a girl remembers for the rest of her life. He looked into my eyes as I held my breath and said, "Stacy, will you marry me?"

I paused only for a brief moment. I didn't know who this Stacy chick was, but I really wanted to get married, and the sparkle on the ring Chris had just pulled out of his pocket was bouncing off the blazing summer sun like a kaleidoscope. Just a quick glance and I could see right away: platinum band, one carat, round, near flawless. In other words, a really nice rock.

"Did you want to maybe rephrase that question?"

"Shit."

He asked again, using my correct name this time. It would be a better story to say that I never did find out who this Stacy person was, though it would also be really disturbing, but Stacy is my middle name, and Chris, it turned out, had planned to say my whole name, but being so nervous, he got ahead of himself. Stacy is also the name of one of my good friends, but I prefer to stick to the former explanation for my own mental health.

We set the date for the following May. Chris had no qualms about incorporating Jewish tradition, as long as all he had to do was show up. I had everything under control. Not surprising since I'd been planning this wedding since I was four years old. The only hitch was finding a bona fide rabbi who would perform an interfaith marriage. I turned to the one person who had an underground network that ran across the entire United States, through parts of Europe, and directly into the Holy Land. My mother set off in hot pursuit, and two days later I had a name.

"So what do you like about one another?" the rabbi asked us as we sat in the living room of his eighteenth-century restored farmhouse, a two-hour drive away.

Chris looked at me. "She has a beautiful smile. It was the first thing I noticed. Plus, she smells like a peach." It was really St. Ives jojoba conditioner, but who was I to correct him?

Then it was my turn. I had my answer ready. "He's kind," I said. Chris rolled his eyes. The rabbi tilted his head, waiting for more. Why does this answer always elicit the same response? Is it so wrong that I just want someone to be nice to me? "And he's intelligent and patient," I added.

We were all set to sign on the dotted line—until he told us his fee, saying, "I've done weddings for free for a variety of reasons, but you two are intermarrying." I was being swindled for marrying a Gentile, but we were out of options, so I cut the check.

The only thing left was to introduce the *machatunim.* We made reservations at a trendy American restaurant in midtown Manhattan. Chris's mother, Nadine, was a refined, well-dressed woman who attended the luncheon with her husband, Mitchell, a retired accountant whom she married when Chris was in his twenties. She had been a hairstylist years ago at the famous Concord Hotel in the Catskills where many city Jews came to summer. This meant that she had experience with neurotic Jewish ladies whose daughters were about to get married.

We took our seats, and my mother waited for us to order the appetizers before pulling out her checklist.

"Which side of the chuppah do you prefer?"

"Either side is fine," Nadine said with a slight shrug.

"What color is your dress? It's better if we don't clash."

"Neutral. Wear what you like."

"We would prefer to have separate family dinners the night before so the bride and groom don't see each other, but we don't want you to feel slighted."

"I don't feel slighted in the least."

"How many people are you inviting?"

"Just us. Maybe a friend or two."

My mother and I glanced at each other. That would never work. How would it look if the groom had no guests?

"Maybe you can come up with some more," my mother suggested.

"Okay."

Nadine was being so agreeable, it was almost as if she didn't care about the Big Day at all, but at least lunch had gone off without a hitch.

On the day of the wedding, as my mother took my arm to walk me down the aisle, a slight breeze lifted my veil and I heard my father's voice: "You've got this, Kabeen." I could almost see his unruly hair neatly combed to one side. He would have been as nervous as I was. I imagined that before leaving me halfway down the aisle for my groom to take me to the chuppah, my father would flash his crooked smile, lingering for a second too long, not entirely sure he was ready to let go. And then, to make me laugh, he'd whisper, "Don't *shtup* too much tonight. Remember, you're still my little girl."

I placed the ring on my groom's index finger, as is tradition. On the inside of his band I had inscribed: "Guardian of My Solitude." Then it was his turn. Inside my band he had engraved: "Forever Your Smile." He smashed the glass and we danced the rest of the night to a fourteen-piece swing band. When he carried me over the threshold to our bridal suite and threw me on the bed, I fanned out my silk wedding dress, poofed up my veil, and embraced the joyful satisfaction that swept over me.

A chance encounter, a fairy-tale romance, and a Great Gatsby–style wedding, and I was on my way to baby-making bliss. Even if *The Ten-Second Seduction* never saw the light of day, it had already fulfilled its goal as a self-help book for at least one person.

5 | Monsters

Weeks Pregnant: 0 to 18

Go to College: Check.
Get Married: Check.

The next step was obvious.

Chris and I had wasted no time. After coming home from one final pre-baby-making trip to Costa Rica just a few short months into married life, I had cornered him in front of the pantry where he was crunching through a box of crackers.

"We're going to make a baby!"

"Right now? I have to go to work."

I swatted him on the shoulder. "Not now. I'm just telling you so you can prepare whatever it is you have to prepare."

"Right. What am I preparing? Do you want me to lift weights? This sounds hard." His head still in the pantry, I could see crumbs forming in a pyramid on the floor.

"Just make sure your boys have a lot of breathing room, okay? Is there enough ventilation under your desk at work?"

"Don't worry, they're safe." He kissed me and headed out the door.

"I'm serious," I yelled after him, but he was gone.

Chris had quit his city job to become a real estate agent, one of the few potentially profitable jobs in our area, but he had been eyeing a lawn and power equipment business that had just gone up for sale and had applied for a loan to purchase it. Real estate took up a lot of time, and he thought that owning a steady business with set hours would allow him to be home more once we had a baby.

On New Year's Eve Chris came home with the flu. I made sure he stayed hydrated and was getting enough to eat because I cared deeply for his well-being, but I'm not going to lie—I was ovulating. I plied him with champagne and made a small attempt at sexy talk, but I could tell I was losing him, and even when our lovemaking reached a fever pitch, I knew his flushed face was because his temperature was rising and not because of my sexual prowess. Luckily, inebriated and sick as he was, Chris was a willing accomplice.

Two weeks later I was standing tall and strong in Warrior One pose during a Sunday morning yoga class, arms reaching to the sky, my lower half grounded toward the earth. Suddenly my legs began to twitch; my flesh tingled. My stomach growled, loudly. People were looking at me. A wave of warmth rushed over me, rising up and enveloping me as though a supernatural force was taking hold. I didn't have to pee on a stick. I didn't scramble to make a doctor's appointment. I knew. After a few more weeks passed, I called my OB-GYN. At the appointment, the nurse marveled at how calm and self-assured I was. I had no questions and I wasn't nervous, which was unusual given my penchant for worrying as a pastime.

I was on a good and steady course, not giving in to my cravings, cutting back on the caffeine, giving up wine and martinis, and maintaining a healthy diet. I even earmarked pages in what I called the "baby bibles" for Chris to read. Every appointment since my first had gone off without a hitch.

At eighteen weeks I came home from a long day of walking around Manhattan with Chris. I was feeling an unusual pain in my lower belly, so I called the nurse. She told me not to worry and that I should wait for my already scheduled appointment the next day to address my concerns with the doctor. Every mother I had confided in had informed me that aches and pains were par for the course, and it almost felt like I was being initiated into a special club.

The exam began in the usual way with the nurse asking questions and taking my blood pressure. When the doctor walked in and said hello, the first thing I noticed was the curve of her lips. They glistened with a red sheen that was painted on so precisely I knew she must touch up her lipstick between patients. I told her about my pain and she asked to examine me, Chris sitting by my side. A few moments later, caught up in my own reverie, I could not make sense of what the doctor was trying to tell me; I could only register the fact that my baby might fall out of my uterus at any moment. My vision began to blur and both Chris and the doctor seemed far away, her voice echoing like she was down a rabbit hole.

I was rushed into an emergency sonogram. Chris squeezed into the corner of the small room. I arched my neck back, compelled to see the screen behind me, as if I could diagnose the problem on my own.

"Wow, um. Okay," said the sonographer, Sherry. She moved her magic wand around my belly and looked at the ultrasound screen. "Let's just measure these." A veil of professionalism swept over her face. I'd seen that look on television shows before, when the nurse lifts the sheets and sees mangled and irreparable body parts.

"What do you see?" I asked, not sure I wanted to know.

"You've got some pretty big fibroids in there. No one ever mentioned this to you?"

"It hasn't come up in conversation." I waited, expecting more, but she said nothing. As she was printing out the scans, the doctor reappeared and said that I had two football-sized fibroids and another tennis ball–sized one growing in my uterus, and because they were so big, they were pressing up against some vital things in there. I don't know if she was exaggerating their size or not, but she had made her point. Oh, and one of those vital things was the baby.

Fibroids are noncancerous tumors that look like big, meaty, bulbous growths. They are a bit reminiscent of that old movie *The Blob* where the amoeba-like alien terrorizes a small town, getting bigger and bigger with every victim it consumes. So my uterus had pretty much become the setting of a horror movie.

I'd had no idea I had fibroids before this moment. I feel it's necessary to clarify this point here because *every single person* I have met since that doctor's appointment, including the doctor, has asked me how it is possible that I didn't know I had fibroids before getting pregnant. But since I had never actually looked inside my own uterus, and no one had ever told me during previous sonograms, I was just as surprised as everyone else to find out. Now I finally had an explanation as to why for the past fifteen years of my life I had to take a pee break every half hour. And yes, I had inquired about this as well but was always shrugged off as women often are when they have medical concerns. In any case I felt momentarily vindicated for all the times I screwed up someone's plans, missed the end of a movie, or caused other people to be late because I had to pee.

My fibroids were so astronomically large that Sherry dubbed them the "Monster Fibroids." In all her years she had never seen such large masses competing with a fetus. The doctor explained that one of the Monsters was pressing against my cervix, and the pressure was shortening it to an alarming degree. The term *incompetent cervix* was bandied about; as if I didn't have enough self-esteem issues, now my cervix was incompetent. That was like five more years of therapy right there. I'd like to lobby for a name change on this one. How about *Independent Cervix That Makes Its Own Decisions About Whom And What It Will Support?* All we need to do is throw in *hostile uterus*, another offensive medical term, and between the two, we'd have the workings of a perfectly dysfunctional marriage. Whatever we chose to call it at the time, the doctor's diagnosis said it all: "There's a good chance you won't be able to support a full-term pregnancy. You'll be tremendously lucky if your baby makes it to twenty-four weeks."

I turned to Chris, who had been sitting quietly as if trying to teleport himself out of the room, and our eyes connected. The color had drained from his face. His full lips formed a flat line but then pursed up on one side. It was too much to bear witness to, and so I averted my gaze. I almost wished he'd scream, get up, ask all the questions, so I wouldn't have to.

I turned back to the doctor, focusing again on her mouth. I no longer saw the rest of her face, just those stop-sign-red lips delivering bad news. Dr. Lipstick was so nonchalant, talking as though she were providing the day's weather forecast, that when I glanced at Chris again he had an expression of utter hatred for this woman. He brought his hands, palms together, up to his mouth and began tapping his fingers.

I was eighteen weeks along, hardly showing my baby bump. The heaviness in my belly was intense, but I couldn't distinguish the physical pain from the emotional. Her words became a jumble as I flashed back to the wintry morning when I had told Chris I was pregnant, a few short weeks after New Year's Eve. The cars were swooshing by on our unplowed road. Standing before him in the kitchen as he was about to pour his cereal, I whispered in his ear, "We planted a seedling." Chris stopped mid-pour, put down the cereal box, and pulled me toward him. We held on to each other's arms and jumped up and down like two kids out for summer recess.

"Already? That fast?"

"One and done, baby."

Grinning, he hugged me. "I didn't think it would be that fast." My normally quiet, reserved husband twirled me around the room and dipped me. We both laughed, shocked and giddy.

But in the doctor's office, with this news, and the way it was presented to us, that memory in the kitchen didn't seem to belong to us anymore. Those were different people full of hope and happiness, and I hardly recognized them. So I put that memory in my pocket for now.

"I don't like her," Chris said dryly when the doctor left us alone, wrapping his arm around me as I got up from the table. I just stared back at him. It was one of the very few times in my life I had ever been speechless.

I threw on my overpriced maternity jeans, embarrassed now that I had spent so much money on this splurge. "I thought I was doing everything right," I mumbled, grabbing my purse.

"You didn't do anything wrong," Chris replied.

Dinner plans forgotten, we drove home, my husband's strong hand holding my thigh.

I wanted to call my father. He would tell me what to do, how to feel, and we would come up with a plan to outsmart the Monster Fibroids. But he wasn't here, and I felt the hollowness of it.

Chris and I woke up early the next morning, limbs entangled. "It'll be okay," he reassured me as he prepared breakfast, urging me to eat. I barely spoke, trying to take a bite of toast.

We drove over an hour to Poughkeepsie to see a specialist. Doctors have a strong need to cover their asses, so the first doctor requested a second opinion. Dr. Lipstick insisted this specialist was the best in the area, and all high-risk pregnancies were referred to him. *High-risk.* It was a term that lingered in the air, like the remnants of an exploded star that can never be pieced back together.

When we were first told a specialist with advanced-tech ultrasound equipment was the next step, I saw money swirling down the toilet. I knew it wasn't what I was supposed to think about, but we had crappy insurance with a high deductible, and specialists tend to charge 250 bucks just to shake hands. It seemed unfair, since I was the one who had to take off all my clothes below the waist; maybe for 250 smackers, the specialist should have to take his clothes off instead. And then, if I liked what I saw, we could go from there.

Dr. Specialist's technician took a fancy picture of my uterus. I could tell that the tech was trying hard to keep her professional demeanor while looking at her screen, but she, like Sherry the sonographer the day before, was horrified. The Monster Fibroids, it turns out, were bigger than the baby.

Dr. Specialist floated in. A gust of wind drifted across the room and the temperature dipped slightly. It was a $250 entrance if I ever saw one. I was almost disappointed to see that his feet did indeed touch the ground. He took off his black-framed glasses and tapped one of the chrome arms against his teeth as he looked over the sonogram pictures. Then he explained to us that eventually there would be a battle of wills when the Monsters would try to suck the blood supply away from the baby, and because the baby was, well, a baby and not a mutant growth, he or she would likely win. (He forgot to mention the excruciating pain this would cause the host uterus.)

The end of this appointment held out more hope than the one the day before, but it wasn't even close to the miracle we had been looking for. We were told that although the largest Monster was pressing against my cervix, and also the baby's head, my cervix was not in as much danger of effacing as Dr. Lipstick had thought. Still, it was a precarious situation, and the message was clear: lie down for the next five months and don't get up. Ever. Well, at least not until the baby starts to crown.

6 | The Pregnant Pause

Week 18, Plus One Day

On the way home from seeing Dr. Specialist that beautiful May afternoon, we stopped at a diner to pick up grilled cheese sandwiches. Cheese and bread were on the short list of foods that didn't make me toss my cookies. I reclined the seat of the Honda as much as I could to take pressure off my lower belly. The pain was becoming more severe by the hour, like a stack of bricks bearing down on my cervix. Chris's hand remained steady on my lap, providing me with quiet reassurance that we were in this together. But I could feel a deep chill creeping over me, settling tight and heavy in my chest, even as rays of sunshine bounced off the hood of the car. It was as though I were in a strange vortex where the warm sun couldn't reach me.

At home we ate the sandwiches on our deck overlooking the Shawangunk Ridge, while Satchie Red, our year-old wrinkly shar-pei, sensing something was amiss, lay down on my feet. The ridge is a hub for world-class rock climbing, and at the top sits the Victorian Mohonk Mountain House and tower. There was no doubt about it; we had a million-dollar view, but the beauty only amplified my grief. There should've been clouds and thunder, a little wind maybe, even some garbage strewn about. The skies should have opened up and unleashed golf ball–sized hail on the world. But there was none of that, not even the smallest breeze to juxtapose my stirring uncertainty, and so, with no other choice, I chewed in silence, distracted only by the ruby-throated hummingbird sucking at his feeder. I remembered him from the past autumn and fleetingly wondered where he had wintered.

Chris finished up the scraps of his lunch. "The closing was today. I just got a call that it's done," he said.

I had known we were closing on the lawn and power equipment business, which we referred to as "the shop," but it had slipped my mind. "Wow," I said. "That's good news. I'm so sorry you missed it."

"Nah," he waved his hand, "didn't plan to be there anyway. But I have to go now and take care of a few things." He kissed me hard on the head, leaving me on the deck.

When I heard his car pull out of the driveway, I wandered over to the bed, laughing quietly at the idea that a grilled cheese sandwich was my last meal of freedom. I stood there, holding the sheets aside. I put my knee up on the edge, about to climb in. I hesitated. What would it mean for me to get into this bed right now? "For five months?" I whispered, but the words caught in my throat.

Sometimes there is simply no pill or procedure, or anything else. Sometimes it's just you and whatever or whomever you believe in trying to figure out how to get through the next moment. I had a hard time coming to terms with the idea that we couldn't just fix this. That *I* couldn't just fix this. What if I just didn't do it? Would I really lose the baby? What was I willing to risk?

I could ignore the doctor's advice. That's what my father would have done. He'd take his chances. No doctor was going to dictate how he lived his life. Each morning, he sat at the kitchen table with his pack of Newport cigarettes, removing two and hiding them. "I'm cutting back," he'd say. And maybe he did cut back, but not enough, and never for very long. "Do as I say, not as I do," he always told me. But what would he say I should do now?

Would I be judged for not agreeing to become a stationary vessel for this child? Probably. The real question was: How much did I care? I needed more information.

I did what almost any other woman would do in my situation: I dropped the sheets in a crumple on the bed, went over to my desk, and googled the hell out of bed rest. Turns out, information around the pros and cons is gravely lacking, and most research is inconclusive. Some experts go so far as to say that bed rest is unethical. What I did find out is that almost *one million* pregnant women each year are labeled high-risk in the United States. My jaw dropped. I found that statistics vary, but *at minimum* 70 percent of those women end up on bed rest for various reasons, including bleeding, gestational diabetes, preeclampsia, carrying multiples . . . the list is endless. That's at least seven hundred thousand women a year suffering from complications that force them to check out of life as they know it, lie down, and wait. I could barely process what I was reading. Those are a lot of numbers, and behind those statistics are real women spending their daylight hours in a horizontal position for less than tantalizing reasons.

I was left with one question: Was bed rest beneficial, or would it just make me physically and emotionally weaker? The only answer I could come up with was: maybe. Maybe bed rest helps, maybe not. Super. Hundreds of thousands of women a year are on bed rest and only a handful of rocket scientists think it's worthy enough to study this phenomenon? If you really want to cheer yourself up, google "stupid scientific studies" to see where we are focusing our resources instead. One such fact-finding mission makes it official that Spiderman doesn't really exist, but all those needy bed-resting women, screw them. It's not like they're superheroes.

The research I did find suggested that most women are put on bed rest to stabilize their bodies. Otherwise normal activities—lifting groceries, exercising, or going to work—

cause additional strain to an already fragile situation. There are also very real benefits to lying down, besides being officially excused from doing laundry for the rest of one's pregnancy; for example, it increases the blood flow to the placenta and thus can slightly increase the baby's birth weight.

But other studies show that bed rest can be hard on a woman's health. A woman's heart and lungs don't work as well as when she's on the move, making her susceptible to blood clots. It can also take a long time to recover lost muscle mass from being in bed for so long. In other words, these studies are saying that not only does bed rest maybe *not* work, but it can actually make things worse.

My own personal conclusion: this was a waiting game to see if I would miscarry or make it to the finish line. I had been thrust into a race that I had not signed up for. I closed my laptop. After I stood on that glacier in Alaska, I came home and gave up everything I had ever known to start a new life. Now here I was, faced with the opportunity to literally nurture a new life growing inside me even though it would mean giving up my mobility, and with it, my independence. I walked over to the bed and pulled back the sheets, not out of some sense of courage or determination, but out of ambivalence. As both my parents so loved to point out, I never stuck with anything that made me uncomfortable. Commitment issues? Perhaps. Would this really be any different?

Those first few days, Chris marveled at my perseverance, telling everyone how I hopped right into bed and didn't get up. It may have looked like that to the rest of the world, this unsung bed-resting warrior, fighting to keep my baby alive, giving up my free will, but the secret truth was—I wasn't so sure how long I planned to stay there.

7 | Purgatory

Week 18½

I was concerned about what people would think. Lying there, with Ralph Lauren cream-colored sheets from my wedding registry pulled up high over my bulging belly, I'd failed to accomplish what most other women seemed to do naturally, and now I had to confess this to the world. Starting with my mother.

There is a pause before you reveal bad news. You know the other person is still spinning in their own oblivious universe and it's all about to come crashing down. You think about that person, what they're doing, how their life will change. I could envision my mother sitting cross-legged at her desk at the Board of Education, where she had worked as an administrative assistant since I was in the fifth grade, wearing one of those long floral skirts she donned daily, matched with a nice pale-yellow cotton pullover. I wanted to give her another few seconds to finish up her lunch, to enjoy the sun streaming through her office window before I ruined her day. My mother was a natural worrier; it was part of her DNA. This would only switch the anxiety lever into high gear.

"How am I going to tell her, Dad?" I said out loud. He had always been our go-between. I'd hide out in my bedroom and he'd sit her down and casually explain the situation, whether it was about my failing grade in math class or that I had just accidentally smashed her best china platter.

I listened in the stillness, waiting for his words.

"Kabeen, don't panic." It wasn't mind-blowing advice, but it was enough.

I looked around the room. I was safe. My baby was still inside me. And somehow I had to convey that to my mother.

Telling her wasn't going to be easy. Not only because she would fall apart, but because she embraced the Socratic method of acquiring knowledge by question and answer; however, it is rare that she actually hesitated long enough to hear the answer, so it's more like question, answer, same question, same answer, a question that has nothing to do with what we're talking about because she misunderstood the answer, and so forth. This usually continues until we both forget what we were discussing in the first place.

"Mom. Don't panic," I said as soon as she picked up the phone.

"What do you mean don't panic? What's happening?"

"They put me on bed rest," I blurted out. So much for laying the groundwork and easing into the conversation. My father had been so much better at this.

"Whaaat?"

"Fibroids. I have fibroids."

"So, what does this mean?" her pitch rising.

I related the doctor's words.

"Oy, okay," she said.

That was it? *Oy, okay?* This I did not expect.

"You know, you'll do what the doctor says, you'll stay in bed and you'll be fine. I'll call you later."

Who was this woman? Last year I mentioned I had pulled a ligament on the treadmill, and she sent me a list of six doctors along with an article about the dangers of sexual assault while running. Now I have a serious medical issue endangering her grandchild's life and she says I'll be fine? I was still staring at the phone in my hand when it rang.

"I hear you're on bed rest. Mom's having a nervous break-down." It was my brother, Mark.

Now my mother's unusually calm demeanor made sense. That crafty woman had enlisted an informant. "How much does she pay you for information?" I said.

"Tell me what happened."

I hesitated. I wasn't sure of his motives. Though my brother and I had professed to be mortal enemies, we could occasionally hold a truce long enough to have a civilized phone conversation, and once when I was in my early twenties, we even managed to take a trip to Italy together. My father was so skeptical, he took bets with his buddies at the bodega that only one of us would come home alive.

But with my father gone, my brother was one of the only people left that I could still count as family. I spilled the medical details to Mark, and he seemed genuinely concerned. Even so, I wasn't ready to wholeheartedly confide in him. Considering his profession as a social worker, not to mention his procliv-ity for exploring ideas that made me feel bad about myself, I knew that any conversation regarding my feelings around bed rest would be deep; I wasn't ready to *explore* my feelings just yet. Plus, there was always the threat that he would have me institutionalized as a way to torture me in our never-ending game of "I Got You Last."

"Well that sucks," he said when I finished.

"Yeah."

"I promise to run interference with Mom. You just worry about yourself and that teeny-tiny baby." I was both surprised and skeptical, but for now I accepted he meant well.

I made a mental list of close friends I wanted to call, and felt a sharp twinge remembering that Rachel and I no longer spoke. We had bonded on the first day of summer camp at eleven years old when no one would pick us for kickball, and we'd sat on the sidelines talking almost every day. In times like these she always had a comforting religious reference to help me remember that a higher power was in control.

I still couldn't wrap my head around the idea that if my husband had a Jewish mother, Rachel and I would still be close. Shortly after I became engaged, I asked her to find out from her rabbi which days on the Jewish calendar were considered off limits for marriage ceremonies that year. Her response was, "You're not marrying a Jew, so it doesn't matter." She'd told me she wouldn't come to the wedding, but naively I thought she would still share in the joy of planning it. Orthodox Jews will say you can't pick and choose the laws you follow, but all my life Rachel had understood and accepted that I was Conservative, not Orthodox, and this is what we did. She had accepted me eating *treif*, but for her, marrying someone who wasn't Jewish went too far. One of the last things Rachel ever said to me was, "Aileen, I will always love you, but I can't condone this." Those words marked the end of our twenty-year friendship.

I dialed a few of my other friends from the city, repeating the same story over and over, until it became something that I could mold and shape and absorb. I never thought my uterus would be such an interesting topic of conversation, but after the first few calls, I had lost all internal filters. I gave anyone who would listen a tour of my reproductive system. I went on about Sherry and her magic wand, about Dr. Specialist and his grand entrance, even about the shade of red lip color Dr. Lipstick was wearing. But when people asked me *why* I was on bed rest, a nervous jolt shot through my chest. I hated the word *fibroid*—hated hearing it and hated saying it out loud. My Monsters were embarrassing. They were big and ugly and I had grown them. They were my shame. But there was no escaping. I couldn't quit my fibroids like I'd quit Brownies.

I had saved the final call for my friend Watson. He wasn't one to mince words, and I knew he wouldn't sugarcoat my situation. "Hey, worst-case scenario, if you lose your baby, I'll be there for you," he said.

Lose your baby. A feeling of relief swept over me. He had said it and my world was still the same. I looked around to be sure there wasn't a small mushroom cloud rising from the corner of the room.

"Just think of it as bed-rest purgatory. The fibroids are the demons you need to slay to save your baby and come back from the underworld." Watson, a copywriter by day for an elite advertising company, was, by night, an aspiring horror writer.

He'd made me smile, but as we said goodbye, I could feel hot tears welling up in my eyes. I hung up and watched the sun making crystal prism rainbows on the wood floor.

When my father died, I cried on and off for a few days, but then I stopped. I could hear him saying, "Stop yer crying, will ya?" I'd heard it a million times throughout my childhood. When I was five, shooting hoops with him on family day at Brooklyn Day Camp (which inexplicably was in Queens), I lunged for a shot and forgot to let go of the ball, falling to the ground and splitting my knee open. The cut was deep. I probably needed stitches, but my father wasn't about to ruin his weekend with a trip to the ER. As my mother tended to me, my father admonished me to stop crying. I didn't understand it; I was physically bleeding and the man was yelling at me. He couldn't stand my vulnerability. One day he wouldn't be here to tend my wounds, and he needed to be certain that I could pull myself together without him.

After he died, I didn't want to let him down, so I just decided that I was over his death, and I refused to mourn anymore. Yet, I couldn't move forward. I began seeing a therapist who looked me in the eye and said, "Your father died. You have a right to be sad."

"I do?" It had never occurred to me that it was my right to feel sad. He would think I was weak, and after his death I had to prove, more than ever, that he hadn't wasted his time trying to mold me into a strong woman.

But what about now? Was I allowed to mourn this? And what exactly was I mourning? The possible death of my child or something else? If this child in my belly died, I knew I wouldn't have the courage to try for another. I had wanted six kids, but maybe I'd never even have one.

"Then what, Dad?" I said out loud. "Then can I cry?"

"Worry about it when it's time to worry," I heard him say.

Was it a time to be strong and buck up, or was it a time to fall apart? Without my father there to yell at me, I fell apart.

Chris was at a loss as to how to help me, and I wasn't ready to share my complicated web of emotions with him. What if he couldn't handle it?

Three days into bed rest, he stood next to me while I lay sprawled across the bed, the back of my hand placed lightly on my forehead as though I were a young nineteenth-century debutante recovering from a fainting spell. If I was going to be forlorn, I might as well be dramatic.

"Can I get you anything?" he whispered, fluffing the pillows.

"No." It was a barely audible squeak. I thought I'd lie down, take a few days, and see what happened. Instead, I was hit with a hormonal roller coaster of despair.

"I don't know what to do for you. Work is crazier than I thought it would be. I can't be here. Today I was trying to explain to this lady that her tractor wouldn't be ready for at least ten days and she started yelling about . . ." He trailed off when he saw my face. "Well, never mind," he said, his lips pressing together in a straight line. He sat down on the bed next to me, hand tentatively touching my leg, as if I might shatter. His eyes were dark and his movements stiff; he was nervous. Then he got up and walked into another room. I needed help. There was only one course of action left: it was time to call in the big guns.

8 | The Whirling Dervish and Her Magic Meatball Sideshow

Two days later, my mother stood in the doorway of the side entrance to our home with a fierce determination to set up a meatball operation in my quaint farmhouse.

"Aileen! *Mamaleh*? I'm here!" she hollered.

Chris was grateful for the support and I counted my blessings that he and my mother had a good relationship. He had been carrying the whole load, taking care of the house, catering to my needs, and trying to learn the ropes at the new business. Just that morning he'd received a shipment of the wrong tractors, and the vendor refused to take them back. When my mother arrived, Chris picked her up from the bus stop, marveling that she was a dynamo who knew how to get things done, and he was more than happy to let her take over.

My mother has a lot of energy—as in, maybe, just possibly, more than she knows what to do with—like a wind farm. She is a petite, thin woman with slightly graying hair, who walks with an affected limp when she remembers. It's as if she's practicing for the time when she knows her bones will start aching. The doctors insist that she is in relatively good health and also that her hearing is perfect, and yet she says, "Whaaat?" at least fifteen times during a five-minute conversation. Again, she's practicing. It takes hard work and severe dedication to perfect the old Jewish lady persona.

She comes from a long line of eastern Europeans who cook when there are problems they cannot solve. No matter that there is no scientific evidence to prove meatballs can cure an ailing cervix; there is always hope. Growing up, our freezer was perpetually filled with frozen meat and matzoh balls from various family catastrophes. When I was in fifth grade and my pet parakeet Murphy died, we had so many leftover meatballs that my mother insisted I bring them to school for international food week, only she made me mash them up and add packets of seasoning so they could pass as taco filling. They didn't.

My mother was convinced beyond a doubt that just the right ratio of sauce, meat, and matzoh meal would make the Monster Fibroids shrink away from my cervix. But because I was a vegetarian, she would have to telepathically summon all the wrinkled little old *balaboostas* from beyond the grave to direct the sauce's healing properties into my uterus. It was as good a plan as any.

She stood over my bed with a package of raw meat in her hands that she had schlepped from Brooklyn.

"Where are your meat dishes?" she demanded.

"Good to see you. Hello!"

"Hello. I need to get the meatballs going right away."

"Chris and I aren't kosher, remember? Just choose some dishes."

She scrunched up her face, repelled by the thought.

After Chris and I had gotten engaged, I had broached the subject of keeping kosher; he'd responded, "So your dishes are kosher, but you're not?" That was the first time I had really thought about it. The intent of keeping kosher isn't that your house is kosher; it's that you're kosher. So why then was there an entire sect of Brooklyn Jews who kept a kosher home but ate bacon (never ham, sausage, or pepperoni) once they left the front stoop? To outsiders, I could see how it looks like a big heap of hypocrisy, but Conservative Jews draw these arbitrary lines based on centuries of tradition, with the occasional modification. My mother sums it up best, saying, "Listen, we do what we can. If God judges, it's between me and him." So basically I had been educated in some of the rules of Orthodoxy and followed them in a way that blended tradition and faith but still allowed me to decide what worked best for my family. Now, my mother, being more conservative than I, was standing over my bed holding two pounds of raw meat, trying to figure out how she was going to cook kosher meatballs in an unkosher house without going straight to hell.

"I'll figure something out. Maybe I'll boil your pots with salt first," she said, going back to the kitchen. That's not a legitimate way to make pots kosher, but hey, we do what we can.

My mother excelled at cleaning, organizing, doing laundry, and scolding me every time I moved. I was to stay stock-still so as not to inadvertently shift the contents of my uterus in the wrong direction. But the cooking, ah, now that was a show worthy of an arena. Pots and pans were struck together with passionate gusto in one shrill crescendo after another—my mother's Meatball Concerto. As a child, I would awake from a sound slumber to the banging, clanging dissonance of eggs for breakfast. I used to think a lack of cabinet space made her pull and push and make a ruckus to get a pot out of the pantry. Only when she began doing this in my relatively spacious kitchen did I realize this noisemaking was her way of summoning the cooking gods and informing them that the food-making ritual was about to commence. Chris grabbed his bag, waved goodbye, and left for work.

When we began our renovations on the master suite, which was really just our bedroom, the nursery, and the laundry room, we had to temporarily relocate our bed. We moved it into the oldest and darkest part of the house, the formal living room. I could just see the kitchen from this vantage point, and I watched as my mother prepped the meat, whirling around like a dervish, throwing wet paper towels against walls, the sink, and even the refrigerator handle in an effort to both cook and clean at the same time, splattering food on the backsplash, and chopping up carrots so fast and furiously that I'm pretty sure I saw specks of blood flying through the air.

Once the cooking was complete, the next part of the ritual began, and I watched as my mother packed everything in Ziploc bags . . . even the wet paper towels. I pulled myself deeper under the covers and rolled my eyes. They were, after all, the only thing I was allowed to move.

"How are you doing, heh? I'm cooking." She was holding up a ladle in her left hand.

"Yes, I heard."

"You heard? You didn't smell? Doesn't it smell delicious?"

"Yes, it smells delicious. Ma, I'm bored and worried."

"You're bored? I'm running around like a chicken without a head and you're bored?" She turned back toward the kitchen. "So, be bored, it's okay," she called out. "I'll tell you what, we'll worry about your feelings later. Just don't die and it will all work out." She gestured with the ladle as she headed for the stove.

Not bad advice, really. Of course, until then I hadn't really thought about dying. But my family does not mince words. We are card-carrying members dedicated to the tenets of tough love.

"You wanna complain? Call your brother," she shouted as she stirred.

I watched my mother dancing about the kitchen, wishing she could just sit still for five whole minutes.

By 10:00 that evening, Chris still wasn't home and I was getting worried. I knew he had work to catch up on and that he probably needed a break from being my caregiver. But he hadn't been in touch all day, and I wondered if he was staying away because of me—because this was all too much. After all, he might lose his baby, too. As my mother headed toward the guest room holding a potato peeler, I stopped her. "Mom, you think Chris is okay?"

She stood at the edge of my bed. "He's probably nervous. He'll do the best he can." She pointed the peeler in my direction. "Look at your father. He was scared of everything, starting with the day we got married."

"What? He was one of the bravest people I ever knew," I said.

"Yeah, right."

"Give me one example of when Dad wasn't brave."

"Our wedding night, and pretty much every day after that."

"What are you talking about?"

"He left me in the hotel room on our honeymoon."

"That's not true."

"It is true. He went to the casino all night. Didn't see him until the next morning."

"What are you talking about? And where are you going with that potato peeler?"

"He couldn't believe what he had just gotten himself into. This is my peeler. I'm putting it in my bag."

"You brought your own peeler? I don't believe you about Dad."

"Listen, when I first met your father, I thought he was complicated and mysterious. But he wasn't. He masked his fears with indifference, so nobody knew. Maybe that sounds like someone else you know?"

"Who?"

"Who do you think?"

"Chris? You don't know Chris very well, and it sounds like you didn't really get Dad either."

"Could be. But I doubt it. What, you think your dad was perfect? I know, I know, I'm the bad one. That's okay. Respect the dead, punish the living."

"How am I punishing you? If that's true, what was Dad so afraid of?"

"Do you want a list? He was afraid one of us would die. That he'd have to be in charge or make decisions. He was afraid to change your diaper. *Schvitzed* buckets until we switched from pins to Velcro tabs."

"No way?" I questioned. My mother was poking some serious holes in the tapestry I had woven of my father's life.

"Chris will come around, or not. I waited a long time for your father to." She began walking away. "Your peeler's no good," she called out.

"So many questions, Ma!" I called after her. She peeked her head around the corner.

"What, you want to know all my secrets?"

"Yes, I do."

"Not right now, I have to eat; it's so late already." The truth was, sure, I wanted to know her secrets, but really I wanted to know my father's.

Chris finally came home around midnight and fell straight into bed, with little explanation. My mother kept so busy that we didn't have another opportunity to talk about my father or Chris again before she had to head back to Brooklyn. I knew how lucky I was to have her on my team, despite the chaos she brought with her, so I told her that I'd look forward to her coming back in about two weeks if she could manage it. We would be okay. At least until we ran out of clean clothes and food. She agreed, promising to call eighteen times a day to make sure I was getting all the rest I needed.

9 | Operation Redecoration

Week 20

Chris found me lying in bed in the dark with dried tears across my face when he came home that evening. I was in a funk, and there was only one way out. If there was ever a time for a shopping spree, this was it.

We were going to need frilly pillows. If you're surrounded by pillows, bad things can't happen. Whenever I feel especially anxious, I stroll through the linen department at Macy's. What could possibly go wrong in a placed filled with plush comforters and soft towels? While I searched online for accoutrements, I asked Chris to collect as many throw pillows as he could find, along with the gold silk sheets we had gotten for an engagement present and rarely used because they made him slide off the bed and hit the floor in the middle of the night.

"Is there going to be room for me with all of these?" Chris said, holding five pillows piled high in shades of purple and cream. He arranged them around me as though they were crib bumpers, then picked up day-old drinking glasses from the nightstand and brought them into the kitchen while regaling me with tales of a customer who wanted to exchange a tractor the shop didn't sell.

I lay there running my fingers over the soft satin pillows, trying to pay attention to his story, but my mind began swirling like a cyclone picking up debris: *trimmers, baby, customers, fibroids, tractors, cervix.* My chest clenched around my heart. The pounding in my ears drowned out Chris's words. I wiped my forehead with the back of my wrist and cold sweat stained my sleeve. *How could people worry about tractors when I might lose my baby?* The room seemed smaller. Suddenly I felt as though I were being buried. Buried under the burden of keeping this child inside me from vanishing. And then I was far from my body, watching myself reach out for a baby that was floating farther and farther away from me. Its small, pink fingers grasped at the air as it drifted, receding until it finally disappeared. "Stop it," I said out loud, looking around the room to ground myself and calling off objects in my head: *Windowpane. Fireplace. Ceiling crack. Sunlight. Breathe.* So much for my frilly pillow theory. I knew I was on the verge of plummeting into a dark place.

"So I told the guy he's clueless—hey, you okay?"

"Yeah, sorry. I just, I don't know," I said, turning away.

"One second. I forgot something." He left the room but quickly returned.

"I found this for you. Thought you might need it." It was my tiara. The one I used to wear while writing *The Ten-Second Seduction.* He placed it on my head. "You'll always be my queen."

If I looked at him, the tears would become a torrent. Instead, I picked up my laptop and pointed to the computer screen. "This pillow is cashmere. I think it goes well with the wood paneling," I said, blotting my cheek with my palm, hoping he wouldn't notice.

"That's the beauty of wood paneling. It goes with everything." Chris pushed my tiara so that it was resting crooked atop my head. "Go ahead and buy it," he said.

I smiled, dropping the pillow in my virtual cart. Scrolling for fancy items reminded me of my first Christmas with Chris's mother and stepfather in New Jersey. That was the day Nadine had invited me into her world of luxury. I had never seen so much decadence in a suburban split-level ranch. From the King Louis XIV Bed and Breakfast Room to the hard eighteenth-century high-backed sofa that looked like it could double for a torture device in the living room, I was unsure where to place myself among the finery. I maneuvered my body into a corner between an ancient Japanese vessel and an abstract painting, where I awkwardly leaned, not sure what to do with my hands, all while wondering where they kept the tchotchkes and family photos. Dinner for four was served buffet style on gold-trimmed china placed upon woven lace—not the "fancy" Dixie plates thrown on a vinyl tablecloth with service for eighteen that I was accustomed to. We discussed rare winter flowers and the Victorian period piece adorning the table—a large crystal bowl held aloft by the outstretched arms of gold-plated vestal virgins. I had thought it was a glorified candy dish. Nadine called it "The Elkington," and when her husband asked how much it cost, her response was, "Not much. How is the ham, dear?"

Dessert was a delicate cheesecake spiraled with fruit and berries—not dried pound cake and sliced cantaloupe. Afterward we gathered around an artificial tree bedecked with ornamental figures from Louis's court, and Nadine presented me with both a Flow Blue dish and purple elbow-length cashmere gloves. The dish looked like it had been taken from a huge collection in her curio cabinet and came with a card that read, "English, circa 1850." A lovely gesture, but at the time it didn't exactly go with my pull-out futon and three-way lamp from the Flatbush Avenue schlock store. The gloves on the other hand, well, I'd bet anything they were from Saks where she currently worked as a hairstylist. As soon as I glided that baby-soft cashmere across my cheek, Nadine had won my heart. Her extravagance was an art form, and though a boudoir straight out of Versailles wasn't in my budget, I now hoped to emulate her by decorating my space with pretty things.

The next day, we moved from pillows to furniture. I wanted to bed rest not just in our bed in the living room but also on the sofa bed in the family room, so I could have a change of scenery. But there was a hitch. If we pulled out the sofa bed in its current position, I'd be staring at the wall instead of the windows with the view.

"Can you please switch the couches in the family room?" I asked my husband.

"What?" Chris had a habit of saying this when he didn't want to do something, as if I wouldn't repeat it and we'd just forget the whole thing. He didn't like change. His memories were rooted in each piece of furniture, every knickknack stuffed in cobwebbed corners.

"It's easy."

"You want me to rearrange the furniture?"

"You want me to stab myself in the eye because I have to stare at a wall for the next five months? Think of the blood, the police investigation, and then of course we might ruin these lovely couches . . ."

"Nothing can ruin these couches. They're practically titanium." They were low-backed 1970s brown velour numbers inherited from Chris's dad along with the house.

After I promised he could switch them back at a later date, Chris acquiesced, swapping the couches and opening up the sofa bed, which led to a dust storm and a solid find of three dollars in change, a small notebook, and a remote control for a television set we didn't own. In the middle, there was a huge stain. Bodily fluids? Blood? Cheap whiskey? Who knew?

"Fit for my queen," Chris said with a goofy smile as he wiped the dust off the mattress and patted it, inviting me to try it out. I attempted to mask the disdain spreading across my face. "Ah, the queen sneers," he said.

I tapped the tiara on my head and winked. Once the sheets were on, I settled in and looked around from my throne. No, my stage. I was a performance artist now.

The first thing I noticed from this new angle was how steeply the floor sloped. If you threw snow on the shag carpet you could call it a bunny hill and charge admission. The pine ceiling and walls made the room look like a fancy shipping container. Not quite what I was going for in the glam department. I could at least amuse myself with the various patterns of wooden knots and cracks in the old pine paneling as I chalked off my time in bed-rest purgatory. The ceiling was like a Rorschach test: sometimes the knots looked like butterflies and fairies, while in dark moments they were demons and baby-eating zombies. The windows looking out upon the view of the mountains (my one saving grace) were the old jalousie kind with metal cranks, but all the handles had long since broken off. The only way to get air was to leave the sliding deck door open, which was covered with a silver shower curtain that looked like aluminum foil. Chris insisted it was a scientifically proven way of deflecting the blazing sun that turned the room into an oven during warmer months.

With my space in order and my emotions stabilized, I had to figure out the logistics of other luxuries, like eating. I was tired of waiting for an authorized pee break to get up and grab a snack, and every time I ate, I had crumbs all over my bed. There was only one solution: tailgating.

I sent Chris down to the Basement of Death and Despair, a place so named because not only was it dark and damp, but it was where we kept the gigantic wolf spiders, creatures the size of my hand that barreled forth wielding their spindly legs like samurai swords. Chris's mission was to find the small blue and white cooler we used for picnics at the private waterfall behind our house. I asked him if he would pack it full of beer each morning, but he refused to be an accomplice to fetal alcohol syndrome so I settled for a few minimally processed, relatively edible food-like options. Suddenly I had my own stage and someone was bringing me meals in bed. Things were looking up.

In truth, due to morning sickness, my diet was limited to two starchy foods (kaiser rolls and Cheerios); one type of unof-

fending vegetable (carrots); and two proteins (fresh mozzarella cheese and cashew nuts). Luckily, most of these fit easily
into mini Ziploc bags. I knew this would make Chris's weekly
grocery shopping trips a snap. But on the first day of this
experiment, it was clear that he had a difficult time remembering to put all these ingredients into bags and then place
them into the cooler. Even more difficult, it seemed, was to
master the closing mechanism on the bags so that the contents
didn't spill out. Chris was in a frenetic rush each morning,
and filling my cooler was just one more thing he was going
to have to do before heading off to work for another day of
lawn mower drama.

On the second day of the cooler experiment, deeply involved
in a television episode of *Barefoot Contessa*, I reached for the
Cheerios and the bag popped open all over my growing belly.
Like a zoom flume, they slid down my body, lodging under my
back and between my legs.

My dog, Satchie Red, taking no pity on a convalescent and
being the fine opportunist her species demanded, pounced
onto the sofa bed, and suddenly we were very intimate as she
searched for Cheerios in unmentionable places. With a growl-
ing sneeze, shaking her head, she began swiping her front
paw along the mattress as if to say, "May the best bitch win."
The race was on, and we both squirmed and scrounged for
Cheerios, seeing who could get them in their mouth the fast-
est. She may have been born with better hunting skills, but I
was blessed with thumbs. Just as I thought I'd proven myself
the superior species, I picked up a Cheerio, popped it in my
mouth, and with grotesque awareness realized that the little
beast had already chewed it up and spit it out.

Understanding that these actions were beneath her, she
refused to meet my gaze. Satchie Red was, after all, a shar-pei
of Westminster lineage—her father had won Best in Breed. But
now she had been reduced to a common mangy mongrel. I

guess the fact that the cooler was on the floor, technically her territory, made the food inside it fair play.

Out of sheer necessity, I added one more game-changing accessory: a tray table. This was my saving grace. Seriously, if there was a fire, I'd save my wedding pictures and this tray table. The tray table itself is an epic invention, and mine came with the addition of a little side pocket to hold small items, which brought the entire contraption to a whole new level of brilliance. This side pocket would spare me hours of trying to find my remote in a sofa bed full of pillows, books, magazines, and food wrappers. I owed my life to the designer of that side pocket.

Satchie Red's animal instinct told her I was weak, and as the days went on, I became paranoid that she was contemplating eating me to thin the herd. If I kept my food on the tray table, we were fine, but if I reached over or ruffled the blankets, she turned her head ever so slowly and stared me down, her upper lip quivering.

"What? You think you have it tough? How many dogs get to eat out of a cooler every day and lounge around on a cashmere pillow? Cut me some slack."

I knew it was tough for her. Satchie Red—whose full name was Aka Satchmo Redstone Princess of All Things Purple Divine and Serendipitous Rotten Sauerbraten, named partially for the great Louis Armstrong and for the red stripe down her back, among a multitude of other situations and incidents, including a bad date I had years before—was my first baby. She was only six weeks old when we brought her home, just a few short months before our wedding. I cuddled her in my arms most days, and when she couldn't settle down at night, I sang the alphabet song to lull her to sleep. Now I could no longer play with her like I used to or take her for hikes along the ridge. I guess we all had some major adjusting to do.

I was ready to settle into bed rest, but there was one final item I was still missing: lip gloss. This tiny tube of happiness has gotten me out of many sticky situations, and once it even got me a few extra cable channels. I wasn't going anywhere, but that didn't mean I had to look like I had no place to go. My lips were the only part of me that wasn't gaining weight, so I planned to show off the assets I still had. Even if I was miserable, I could still look dewy. Besides, the UPS guy, who reminded me of Charlie Chaplin with his bushy eyebrows and funny little mustache, might stop by.

I went on Amazon to see if I could order some lip gloss . . . in bulk. By the time I was done with my spending spree for the week, it totaled more money than I cared to think about. Was I overcompensating, trying to cover up my pain and creeping depression with sparkles and sheen? Maybe. But this was the time to indulge. I looked around the room. This was my stage and I was going to perform amazing feats of bed-rest magic here.

10 | Dos and Don'ts and Don'ts

Week 21

Surely no one expected me to really just stay in bed *all* day. Three weeks after first pulling back the sheets, we headed out to my OB-GYN appointment, where I would try to clarify what *they* meant by "bed rest." Maybe (hopefully, dear God) I had misunderstood. There must be more to it than staring at the wall.

The car ride was exceptionally riveting after being stuck in the house for so long. The scent of the purple lilacs, the loud hum of yellow construction cranes idling around a new community project, people on the walkway along the main drag sporting spring jackets, colorful yoga pants, and a rainbow of tank tops—it reminded me of the first time I turned on our brand-new technicolor TV after my family upgraded from an old black-and-white in the seventies.

As I waited my turn to be called, I convinced myself that Dr. Lipstick would say it was perfectly fine to go to the gym for light yoga once a week. Maybe she would tell me it was all a mistake; I wouldn't have to fully commit to bed rest at all. I'd be back to my normal life in no time.

Chris waited while I went for yet another sonogram, and we met in the examining room afterward.

I slipped into a fresh paper robe and jiggled my shoulders. "Sexy, no?" I said.

His eyes lit up as he laughed. "You wear it well."

I hoisted myself onto the table, swinging my legs while I waited. Ten minutes later, Dr. Lipstick strolled in wearing black heels with red soles. *The lady has Louboutins.* Chris, still holding a grudge, turned away, pretending to read a poster about human papillomavirus. I ogled the doctor's pumps, following her stockinged legs up her tight yellow frock to her glossy lips. *That's got to be Chanel red.*

"Looks like your fibroids are continuing to grow. We just have to hope for the best."

"Can you remove them?"

"We can't do anything about them now. That's a discussion for another time, when you're no longer pregnant."

My shoulders slumped. Chris's back stiffened.

She pointed to a dark blob on the sonogram. "That's your cervix. It's not supposed to look like that. You can see the fibroids compressing it."

This did not make me feel attractive. I pictured the Monsters jelly-like, with hair and teeth, similar to the talking mucus on those famous decongestant commercials. I turned my head to see Chris's eyes boring into the poster.

"Can I exercise?"

She tilted her head, her expression saying, "You poor, misguided girl."

Can I at least try on your Louboutins? I thought desperately.

"Do whatever you can to alleviate the pressure. Try lying flat on your back with your hips up." I eyed her with what was becoming my patented look of disdain. Did she not realize that this was the exact position that had gotten me into this mess in the first place? "Or lie on your left side to take pressure off the vena cava. This is the really big vein that brings blood from your lower body back to your heart. The bigger the uterus gets, the more likely it is to put pressure on this vein."

Great. With all my other issues, now I had to worry about pissing off the vena cava.

As she turned to leave the room, I called her back. There was one more thing I needed to be 100 percent clear about. I locked eyes with her, then cupped my hand over the right side of my mouth, whispering loudly while pointing into my hand at Chris, "What about a little bit of sex?" I joined my palms together, making the universal sign for prayer. She pursed her lacquered lips to one side and gave a short, negative headshake.

At home I stacked two pillows under my butt and put my legs up the wall. When my back started cramping up, I put a yoga block under my sacrum to maintain a slight inversion. Still not ideal. I looked around for some other creative aids and fondly recalled the days when props + bed = fun.

For the rest of the afternoon, I busied myself writing down a list of bed-rest dos and don'ts. Even this simple task proved almost beyond my capability. The pen kept making holes in the paper I was holding over my belly and my writing was illegible. I grabbed a magazine to pad the paper and tried to write holding it up over my head, but the ink stopped flowing. I rolled onto my side, and my arm began aching. I then tried balancing the tray table over my growing belly, but that, too, was cumbersome. I finally positioned the table to my side, and though I had to turn my head, it seemed to work.

The Do List was easy:

> *Do eat in an awkward reclining position*
> *   with two pillows under your hips*
> *Do hold your pee as long as possible so you don't get up too often*
> *Do shower for only two minutes a day*
> *Do remember to* BREATHE

Alarmingly, the Don't List proved to be much longer:

> *Don't walk*
> *Don't drive*
> *Don't cook*
> *Don't exercise*

Don't do laundry
Don't lift anything
Don't sit up
Don't go anywhere
Don't have panic attacks
Don't HAVE SEX

I knew that my sex life was going to change with pregnancy; I just didn't count on it coming to a sudden halt. This was not good. Our marriage was young, and physical intimacy was a big part of it. Would Chris still find me attractive? Would we have to limit ourselves to cuddling? Would that be enough, or would bed rest cause an irreparable rift?

I tried not to think about it, but I had so many questions: Would I ever be desirable again? And what about my friends? Would they forget about me? Had anyone told Rachel? I had hoped that word would get around through the yenta network in the synagogues across Brooklyn and she'd at least send an email with well wishes. Normally Rachel would have visited with me, brought me nosh and a few nights' worth of dinner. She would have made me laugh and told me it was all in God's hands, and it would have both comforted and annoyed me because I couldn't fix it. I pressed my lips together and looked down. I knew better. She had moved on. I wondered if she ever reached for the phone or thought, *Oh, I can't wait to tell Aileen,* before remembering that she couldn't. I sat with the sting of it.

I needed to get up, prove that I still had some autonomy, however small. With no place to go, I settled on walking to the mailbox to retrieve the mail. Maybe there would be a package, or a letter. Our mailbox, while not very far from our house, was across the street. It required shoes and a reasonable amount of clothing, both of which I had been lacking. I swung my legs to the floor. Sat up. Stayed there. Okay, I couldn't have sex, but mail was kind of fun. I ran my toes along the shag carpet. Feeling rebellious, I hoisted myself to a standing position. Just the kitchen. I could decide from the kitchen. I mean, I wasn't going to kill my baby by getting the mail. I made my way to the side door, but a dull pain in my lower belly stopped me, driving me to a squatting position on the yellowing linoleum floor. The Monsters protested.

"Get back into bed. Whaddaya, outta ya mind? That's my grandbaby!" My father's voice came through loud and clear. Defeated, I squat-waddled back to the sofa bed, cradling my belly with my forearm.

"You would have made some grandfather," I said, looking up and shaking my head. I imagined him sitting on the floor watching ball games, shouting at the television, and during commercials, teaching his grandchild blackjack or playing tricks on Grandma, maybe even sneaking the kid a swig of Heineken. For the first years of my life, that was the man I knew.

Then, one morning when I was getting ready for kindergarten, I saw him sitting at the kitchen table, his steaming coffee filled to the brim as he wrote on a piece of paper.

"Why aren't you at work?" I asked. He was a buyer in the garment district and usually long gone by the time I awoke.

"That's done. Yosh and I are going to be PIs. Do you know what that is?" He told me that he and his best friend were quitting their jobs to open a detective agency. Of course, even I knew that he couldn't find two matching socks in a dresser drawer, let alone clues to a real mystery, but he was optimistic, and I thought the plan sounded fabulous. My mother, probably not so much.

Now I wondered, how could he quit a good job for a wild scheme when he had little mouths to feed? It sounded selfish to take such a risk, especially with no experience and no connections as a private investigator. Here I was on bed rest, struggling to find a way to continue working, temporarily casting aside my own basic needs, including the freedom to take a shower, for a baby whose life wasn't even guaranteed, and my dad had quit his job for a pipe dream. I knew there must have been more to the story than I was remembering. He had sage words of advice for me whenever I wanted to make a drastic life change, so surely he wouldn't have given up a lucrative career without reason. Or would he? I had to find out what actually happened all those years ago. I settled in the sofa bed, focusing on my breathing until the pressure of the Monsters in my belly subsided, and called my brother for details I had been too young to understand at the time.

"It's a great story. No one ever told you?"

"I guess I always thought I'd ask Dad. I didn't know we were on borrowed time."

"Well, in the seventies the garment industry was rife with mafia. Things were heating up," he said.

"Dad was not in the mafia. We're Jews."

"You've never heard of the Kosher Mafia?"

"Are you kidding me?"

"They torture their victims by forcing them to eat gefilte fish."

"For years I always thought there were little gefiltes swimming in the ocean."

"Well you're not that smart."

"We're getting off topic," I said.

"Right, so the Kosher Mafia is a thing, look it up. I'm not saying this was the Kosher Mafia. I really don't know. I was eight at the time and not up on the affiliations of organized crime families. But the fact remains that our daddy was possibly involved in some shady dealings. A few months before he quit his job, he was arrested."

"But the charges were dropped," I said. I had a vague recollection that my father had been arrested and that nothing had ever come of it, but we had never been allowed to discuss it.

This was our one big family secret, the only piece of information the Weintraubs had not put out there for the world to see. Of all the ways we had hurt one another both physically and mentally over the years, of all the horrible accusations made in the heat of the moment, this was our shame. My father had been taken into a police station and within a few hours was released. How would our family ever recover?

"Yes, the charges were dropped. We'll never know what really happened. But either way, it was time for Dad to move on. Yosh and Dad agreed to quit their jobs and become PIs."

"And Mom?"

"He quit before telling her. What was she going to do? Incidentally, she would have made a better PI than him."

"It's true. You can't pull anything over on that woman." Growing up, Mark and I were convinced that every pigeon in Brooklyn was secretly working for my mother, spying on us and reporting back. If we were late to Hebrew school, she knew. If we were fighting in the streets, we'd get smacked when we came through the door. "So what happened with the PI plan?"

"Yosh died."

That's all the information my brother had. So I called my mother for the rest of the story.

"When Yosh died, our lives changed," she said.

"What are you saying?"

"Your father fell apart. And he never put himself back together."

"How did Yosh die?"

"Very suddenly. Dad never told me the details."

Perhaps it was the first time my father had faced his own mortality. Or maybe it was because he had just quit his job, and now, without Yosh, he was left with nothing. Whatever the reason, he never recovered. He took to the couch and did not get up for the next three years. I thought he was lazy, or that he didn't care about us anymore. Nobody had told me it was because he was wrecked. Now, lying in wait, I knew what it was like to do that same dance with depression. But if my mother had known this, did she try to help him? I asked her as much.

"Of course I tried to help him. I tried everything. But Aileen, you have to want to help yourself. Your father did not want my help, or anyone else's. He had given up."

"Just like that?" I whispered.

"Just like that," she said.

I wanted to be angry at her. I wanted to ask her why she didn't do more to fix him. But my anger was misplaced. She had kids to tend to and a husband who couldn't function for years at a time. She was the one holding it all together.

I don't remember the first time I came home from school to find him curled up on our green velvet, plastic-covered couch. It had become his default position: a Newport burning in the ashtray on the floor while the television blared daytime shows and he dozed in and out of a fitful sleep.

Some days, if I was persistent, he would rally to play a game we had made up. I'd stand in front of him, hands on my hips, blond curls askew. "Just once?" I'd ask. "Nah, you're too big," he'd say. Even the asking had become a game. "Once?" I would plead. "Okay, c'mon, let's go." I'd circle the living room jumping up and down to warm up, and then run as fast as I could, leaping over his body. He'd wrap his thick giant hand around my torso and shove me down behind him, so I was wedged between his back and the couch. Sometimes he'd reach his hand back and tickle me, but mostly I'd stay there for hours while he watched television and slept, drawing imaginary pictures on his back, listening to him snoring with his mouth agape. That was my safe place, even when I was too old for such things and I barely fit. I wanted to be there now, a little girl again, cradled between cold plastic and my father's soft, warm body, my chin resting on his fleshy bicep, watching the rise and fall of his thin plaid button-down shirt as he drew rhythmic breaths, close enough that I could hear his beating heart.

My mother had moved after my father died—each time she opened the front door, the smell of menthol Newports, forever seeped into the wallpaper, flooded her with too many memories. I knew I'd never see that place again.

As I was thinking about how one unexpected event can change the course of a person's entire life, Chris came home from the shop.

"We have enemies," he said.

"I know three people in this town. One of them is you. I haven't had time to make enemies."

"Everybody hated the old owner."

"And so . . . by proxy?"

"Turns out he didn't deliver on a lot of promises. I've had people yelling at me all day."

Buying a local business had been Chris's dream. When the lawn and power equipment shop came up for sale, Chris signed on the dotted line with stars in his eyes, enamored of all the shiny red tractors standing in two neat rows. Now the harsh fluorescent light of reality was setting in. He leaned his forehead against the sliding-glass door and looked out at the ridge as he spoke. "The old owner was less than honest, the place has a bad reputation, and everyone wants their tractors today. No one wants to wait. We're backed up for three weeks." As he repeated the litany of complaints he had heard that day, I wondered how this introverted man I had hitched my future to was going to make nice to all those angry tractor-hungry people, some of whom still owed money to the business.

"Can't you just tell them you'll deliver their equipment when it's finished being repaired?"

"People have an aversion to tall grass."

I reached for my list and wrote:

Don't buy a business with a bad reputation

As a former jiu-jitsu fighter, Chris had developed an almost obscene level of patience. He was calculating; they called him the Sandman because he would wait out his opponent, not going in for the kill until just the right moment. And then he'd take down the guy and put him to sleep before he even knew what had hit him. But I wasn't sure how this was going to translate to lawn mower repair. This business wasn't just some small mom 'n' pop shop as we had thought. Chris had assumed he could hire someone to run it and just check in for a few hours a day. But the reality was that this was a full-on commitment with a huge learning curve for stuff like understanding the subtle differences between a transmission belt and a deck belt, or knowing that Farmer Sheehan can only have her mower delivered on Tuesday afternoons before 3:00 p.m. There were work orders and invoices and endless varieties of grass-cutting paraphernalia—tractors, push mowers, zero-turns, commercial, residential. Yawn.

Given my penchant for shiny objects, it may come as a surprise that my enthusiasm for power equipment wasn't quite as off the charts as Chris's. While I truly wanted to be a supportive wife, in no way did I see myself ever selling tractors.

Once, while we were dating, Chris tried to start me off on a basic ride-on mower. After some cajoling, I mounted the tractor like a motorcycle, pressed the switchy thing, and then nearly flew right off as it throttled forward.

"Shut it off, SHUT IT OFF!" I yelled as the tractor continued to propel onward of its own volition, my arms flailing.

"Hold on, hold on," Chris called out.

"I'M GOING OFF THE CLIFF!"

"You're about forty feet from the hill." He caught up to me and grabbed control of the tractor.

"SHUT IT OFF!"

"Aileen. The lawn mower is off."

"I COULD HAVE DIED. I'M ALMOST DEAD RIGHT NOW." I straightened my shirt, glanced at my watch, and said, "Oh, look at that, it's cocktail hour."

"Maybe we'll try again later?" he called out hopefully. Needless to say, we never did.

Now, here we were, a bajillion dollars in debt, and I was suddenly, very unexpectedly, horizontal. I was out of my comfort zone in this house, with this business. Historically, this was the exact moment I would choose to make my grand exit, fly off on an adventure, change my life, climb a glacier, run. But now I was stuck in my fidgetiness, fighting a battle inside my own skin to stay put. Reality struck hard and fast.

Don't leave

Chris came over to the bed, fingernails black with the day's work, and put his hand on my belly. His gray pants were splattered with oil and a burn had ripped a hole in one of the legs. Even his baseball cap was coated in thick black dust around the rim, beads of sweat glistening on his forehead.

"I got a lot going on," he said. Just then the baby began to tap dance. "I know, little one, I hear you."

"I guess the little one has a lot going on, too. He's growing fast." I put my hand on top of Chris's. For the last few days it had felt like a flutter, and I couldn't be sure, but now there was no mistaking it. "The baby just kicked for you. That's huge."

"It is. The problem is, everything feels huge right now."

"This is good. It means he's hanging in there."

Chris blinked hard. I could see new creases forming around the corners of his blue eyes. He was being pulled in a hundred different directions. A new business, an ineffectual wife, and more debt than we could have ever imagined. I knew what he was thinking: this business could not fail; this pregnancy could not fail. It was that simple. He didn't know where to put his resources, only that he was running out of them fast. How many more cracks could appear before everything collapsed?

Do rob a bank

He sat down next to the couch on the pink-and-blue-striped chair that in no way matched any other object in the room, leaned back, and looked at the ceiling.

"I just don't have time to process everything that's happening right now. Maybe I could drive you to Brooklyn and you could stay with your mom for a while," he suggested.

Wait. Maybe . . .

Do leave?

"I don't know. I'd never be able to go outside. Here I can be on the deck." My mother now lived on the sixth floor of an apartment building.

"How about my mom in Jersey? I'm sure she'd pamper you."

With her keen eye for finery, Nadine did treat her guests well. She was an excellent cook, and she put out the softest towels in the guest bathroom, along with the most decadent shampoos and creams. After the wedding, she and I began chatting more often. She would tell me about her antique finds or a new perfume that had debuted at Saks. She ended every conversation by asking if I needed her to buy anything for the house. It felt genuine, but something in her tone reminded me that our house was old and needed work. I considered what it would be like to have an extended stay in the Louis XIV Bed and Breakfast Room. At first it sounded like a vacation, but without Chris, I knew after a day or two I'd feel trapped in a gilded cage. I'd be even lonelier than I was now. And what if the worst happened? What if I began to bleed? I couldn't bear the thought of being rushed to a hospital, being told my baby was dying without Chris by my side.

I didn't want to be in Jersey, or Brooklyn, and I didn't want to be sent away to convalesce. I wanted to be with my husband. We were a married couple, and that's what married couples do, for better or for worse. Besides that, my mother-in-law didn't understand the seriousness of the situation. As quiet, well-composed Gentiles, Chris's family dealt with life's mishaps in a very calm manner, and I wasn't about to have anything to do with that. They rarely go off the deep end, whereas my family lives on the shores of those uncharted waters.

When I told Nadine that I was now on bed rest, her response was, "Aw, that's too bad. I'm sorry you're not feeling well. Can I call you back? I have out-of-town guests coming and I don't know where Mitchell put the silver. I think it's in the garage." A few days later she sent me a care package. It was a gigantic Slurpee cup that read "There's Big and Then There's Bubba."

Don't send subtly offensive gifts about size to pregnant women

"There is no good solution to this," I said, feeling that Chris might be trying to push my care off on someone else. It would serve him well to take a few things off his plate, but I wasn't something to be delegated.

"We'll get through this," he said.

"I'm sorry I've become just another item on your to-do list."

"That's not fair."

"Well, you're trying to ship me off somewhere."

"I've got one of those big shipping stamps at the shop; we could put it on your forehead."

"That's not even a little funny."

He said nothing.

Another series of kicks stopped me from pursuing the conversation. There would be time to find out what he truly meant. Chris got up from the chair, but I motioned him toward me, pulling his hand onto my belly one more time to remind him of the life we were fighting for.

"This can't be scratched off a to-do list," I said.

"No," he said, and his eyes softened.

As he walked away, I added one last item to *my* list.

Do: Hope

11 | Bras on Fire

Week 22

Scratching off the first full month of bed rest, the bills were piling up, and I woke one morning with an ache that, for once, didn't come directly from the Monsters. It was time to get back to work on my own projects and contribute to our financial well-being. I was lucky to have a long lead time on a book about railroads I was editing for a small independent press, but now the deadline was looming. As a freelancer I could work from anywhere and set my own hours, and it seemed that bed rest shouldn't interfere, but the reality was, I no longer wanted to get out of bed even if I could. I had lost the will to be productive, and like my father at his lowest point, I began sleeping away the day.

Until now I had never gone a week without working. At the age of twelve, I had steady babysitting gigs, and at fourteen I had my first job at Dunkin' Donuts. In college I worked nights and weekends to make the rent. Watching my family struggle with money as my father fell deeper into his own world had instilled a strong work ethic in me. I walked a tight rope, juggling my passion for writing with making sure I could always provide for myself.

Directly out of college, I landed a job on Wall Street, but after a year I began interviewing for a position that wasn't as soul crushing. I turned down an offer at a hedge fund making double the salary to look for a job in publishing. It was a life-changing decision, but I knew that if I didn't get out of the financial world, I'd get sucked in and it would become difficult to walk away from a hefty paycheck. I called my father to tell him, thinking he'd be disappointed that I hadn't seized the opportunity. "I'm so proud of you, Kabeen. Never go for the money; it's not worth it. Sometimes you go for the money and you end up with nothing," he said, surprising me.

But I did long to feel financially secure, and part of the reason I was drawn to Chris was his ambition. Now, with the shop putting us in debt, we were on shaky ground. Luckily, I could allocate funds with the skill of an illusionist. I had learned from the pros, watching my grandmothers clip coupons and scour the racks for deals. But nobody could strike a bargain like my mother. In the late nineties she upgraded our yellow paisley-patterned vinyl dining room chairs with modern cherrywood and real fabric, which to this day are preserved in plastic. She had visited the furniture store so many times, bringing swatches, paint chips, and friends, that the salesman sweetened the deal with a steep discount just to keep his sanity. It was all part of my mother's master plan.

I lay in bed calculating my next steps when the eardrum-bursting shriek of our doorbell jostled me. The only way to stop the ringing was if someone un-jammed it by stabbing the button repeatedly. Satchie Red howled, chasing her tail as if capturing it were the secret to stopping the deafening sound. She thought every person who came through the door was trying to kill us; when that doorbell rang, shoes were shredded, puddles appeared on the floor, slobber went flying against the walls, and yet we did nothing to fix it. "That's the way that doorbell has always been. Good enough for Pop, good enough for us," Chris quipped when I begged him to replace it.

Jackie un-jammed the bell and came in without waiting for an invitation. Flaming red hair, the smell of cigarettes on her blouse, Jackie, close to my mother's age, was the wife of Chris's friend Nan. With one swift snap of her fingers and a firm "Quiet!" she silenced Satchie Red, who ran behind the chair in the corner and whimpered.

"Hi! I brought you a scone." She threw a small paper bag at me.

Even though I had only previously met Jackie at large gatherings, I found her easy to talk to, and because my limited contact with the outside world had caused me to forget social niceties, I wasted no time asking her if she thought I should continue working or put it aside. Part of me was hoping she would give me a pass, tell me I shouldn't work, and instead focus on my pregnancy.

She pointed a long scaly finger at me. "It's a tough decision. How can you focus on editing right now? What you're doing here, in bed, that's important work. But I'll say this: never depend on anybody else, not even your husband." It sounded like she was speaking from experience. "I have children, those rotten bastards, so I know how hard it is to keep it all together. Don't give up on your career. Keep your finger in the pot at all times."

I winced, mostly because she was echoing what I already knew. My income was meager, but it did pay some of the bills, and more than that, it gave me independence.

Jackie took a seat across from the sofa bed and began telling me about her former career as an office manager for an insurance company. She did that to pay the bills, but I also learned that she had been on the front lines of the feminist revolution. She had marched in protest for equal pay, refused to wear a bra for most of the seventies, and liked to quote Gloria Steinem. She left her husband when divorce was rare, to be with her current wife, which at that time had been even more taboo.

"Listen, my wife, she's the breadwinner. But I've got my own thing going on. Make sure you keep your own thing, too. Life changes on a dime. Gotta run. Kisses." Her words were a lot more than I had bargained for that early June morning.

Growing up in a Jewish community, the roles were clearly defined. The husband went to work, and the wife was responsible for keeping the home and raising the children, even if she worked. My friend Rachel had an advanced degree but then chose to stay home and raise her family. When I asked her why she spent all that money on an education, she explained that she did it for herself. I respected that, but while I had a deep-rooted desire to build a home and create a family, I also knew I needed to maintain my career like my own mother had. She had stayed home with me until I was in the fifth grade, but then went back into the workforce both out of necessity and for her own autonomy. Chris's mom went back to work when he was two weeks old. Our mothers didn't have a choice, but now he and I were lucky. When I became pregnant, we agreed that our kid would not experience the loneliness that we'd experienced as latchkey kids. As a freelancer I could be home most days, and with his shop just down the road, Chris would have the flexibility to be there when I couldn't. We knew that most parents didn't have this option and we considered ourselves fortunate.

Now, laid up in bed while Chris worked twelve- to fourteen-hour days, it was dawning on me that I might have to give up my career, at least temporarily. Jackie had validated how difficult it was to check out of life to lie down and wait. This wasn't the Victorian era; women didn't go into confinement when they became pregnant, dropping out of society to hole up in a dark, airless room and magically reappear months later with a baby as if it had been delivered by the stork. We had jobs and obligations, and some of us even had countries to run. We had revolutions to join and protests to organize. I needed to be strong and solid and carry on, despite my failing body. It made me want to get up and burn my bra—metaphorically, of course; lying down gave me a bad case of side boob.

I opened my laptop, trying to balance it on my belly, and began working on the manuscript about railroads I had been editing. It was difficult to get the angle just right and it kept sliding off. I caught it twice, but the third time, when I finally thought I'd figured it out, I got cocky, typing, balancing, and reaching for a beverage at the same time. As the laptop began its slow-motion descent to the floor, I dropped my unsweetened iced tea, drenching my shirt, desperately trying to save the computer from that final thud. I flinched at the sound of it hitting the floor. Propped up on pillows, feeling tea soaking through my shirt, I was going to have to wait to deal with my garments until I was allowed my pee break in half an hour. I sopped up what I could, reached for my laptop, and moved to the dry side of the sofa bed. Thanking the lords of electronics that it rebooted, I twisted onto my left elbow to work, but soon my whole arm was tingling and I was convinced I was having a heart attack. I called Watson in a state of panic.

"Which arm hurts when you're having a heart attack?"

"What? I don't know. The left? The right, I think it's the right."

"My arm is tingling! I'm dying. It's happening right now."

"Why are you calling me, call 911!"

"I don't want to bother them!"

"Take a chill. Sounds like anxiety. Trust me. I've been there." It was true. Watson suffered from levels of anxiety even I couldn't achieve. "Now, why does your arm hurt?" he continued.

"Because I'm lying on it."

"I'm changing my phone number," he said.

"That's not very supportive."

"What's the real issue here? Because we know we're both going to have to deal with it eventually." Watson indulged my angst to a point, but then usually made me cut the crap. Having grown up in the same neighborhood, we understood each other's *mishegas*. We were also both married to people who did not dwell on life's little problems, so we only had each other as we struggled to crawl through those emotional trenches. He was pretty much me, minus the pregnancy hormones.

"Well, if we're going to be rational about it," I said, sighing, "I'm afraid I'll never be able to work again. I can't even juggle a laptop and iced tea, how am I going to work with a baby?"

"Try it; if it doesn't work out, take off a couple of years and then go back. It will still be there."

This sounded very reasonable, which is why I wasn't having it.

"What about the mommy pay gap? It's a thing," I said.

"Do you really make enough money to be concerned about that? You think you're the first person to have to deal with this? You'll make it work, like everybody else." Watson gave it to me straight, and sometimes that was exactly what I needed.

I turned my attention back to the manuscript, working in ten-minute intervals, lying on one side until my arm tingled, then rolling over to the other side. This was not sustainable.

By the end of the day, it was evident I'd have to hold off on new projects. I had already agreed to two others, and once again, here I was, unable to keep a commitment. I emailed my publisher explaining that I didn't feel confident I would be able to work to the standard he expected. He responded with kindness, leaving the door open for me to get back in touch when I was ready.

Filled with guilt and a sense of despair that I had let down yet another person, I looked around the room and took stock; our sofa used to be where Chris and I had long make-out sessions and talked about our future plans. Now it felt like a hospital bed with half-filled cups and magazines piling up. I considered working on *The Ten-Second Seduction*, but it sickened me to admit that my life had changed so drastically. This vibrant, self-proclaimed seductress had been kicked to the curb. I laughed at the thought of a book tour in my current state—my overworked husband wheeling me around on a hospital bed from one signing to the next as I waxed poetic about all my sensuous encounters.

Maybe I had to take a writing hiatus, but this sofa bed was still my office space. I just had a new job description: Legs Closed, Hips Up, Don't Let This Baby Fall Out.

12 | It Comes Down to Blood

I'd always been a firm believer in not having too many places to lounge. It encourages all-around lackadaisicalness. But now that I was to do nothing but lounge, I deserved a comfortable chair in the shade. Unfortunately, my deck was south-facing, and with the temperature heating up, I couldn't even step foot out there without feeling like I had been sucked into Dante's seventh circle of hell.

I sent Chris on a mission to find a deck chair and matching umbrella. The plan was for him to scope out what other patrons were buying and come home with something similar. As I awaited my purchase, I envisioned myself whiling away the days, observing the wildlife. There was the iridescent-green hummingbird who dive-bombed the feeder like a kamikaze fighter when the ruby-throated male hummingbird wasn't around. I bet she appeared svelte and sexy when they were on dates, like the kind of bird who just ate salads but then binged on sugar when no one was watching. I'd tell her that men like chicks who eat. Then I'd commiserate with the robin who was building a nest in the lilac tree that overhung the deck railing. I'd warn her to take one last flight of freedom before settling down to lay those eggs. We would talk about our hopes and dreams and it would be beautiful and serene, and it wouldn't feel like bed rest at all. Hell, it would feel like a fucking Disney movie.

As I was expanding the list of animals I'd capture to ply with unsolicited advice—the woodchuck who took one bite out of every single tomato in our garden; the deer who scratched its antlers against my magnolia tree until it fell over; the sex-crazed rabbits who just needed to calm down—Chris arrived home, arms full and struggling up the driveway.

"This will never work," I said as he tore apart the plastic wrapping and began setting up the new chair.

His shoulders fell. "I looked at ten different chairs. This was the best option."

"It has to recline all the way back. That's the whole point of bed rest. And there's no cushion."

Chris sighed and turned to go.

"The umbrella looks good, though," I shouted after him.

I ordered an umbrella stand online, and after two more trips to the big-box stores, Chris came home with an acceptable chair. My jiu-jitsu fighter was living up to his nickname. The Sandman was still holding firm to his patience. I wondered if my father was this tolerant of my mother's requests when she was pregnant.

Two days later, through the modern miracle of free expedited shipping, the Charlie Chaplin UPS guy was at my door. This rare human contact was the highlight of my day.

"Here you go, Aileen. I need a signature," he said.

"How'd you know my name?" Suddenly this felt creepy.

"It's on the box." He smiled, his brown eyes sparkling below thick brows.

"Oh, right. So, what's your name?"

He pointed at the name tag on his uniform. "Dave."

"There it is," I said. "Well, thanks, Dave."

Dave's arms were tan. I tried to picture him without his mustache. Would it be weird to ask him to put his finger above his lip?

"Everything okay?" he asked.

"My brother has a mustache." I had been locked up for too long.

"Oh. Okay. Well, you have a nice day." He stroked his mustache and smiled before heading back to his truck. Halfway across the front yard, he stopped, turned, and waved. Oh my God, the man thought I was flirting with him, when really I was just a moron.

The next morning Chris set up the umbrella but then left for work without opening it. It was colossal, and it would require more strength and maneuvering than I could muster; how was I supposed to open it—from bed? Years later I would look back at these little communication difficulties and wonder if they were the seeds that sowed greater misunderstandings. At least the cushy chair was there and the deck umbrella was physically on the deck; unfortunately, the only thing it was doing was blocking the view.

The days were long. I pretended the deck was a yacht off the coast of France, and I was waiting for my garçon to arrive with a dry martini. Luckily, every afternoon at 4:00 p.m., there he was, his rugged hands greasy with motor oil. Instead of a martini it was a decadent chocolate or vanilla milkshake. Well, maybe not decadent, but good enough for a broad shackled to her bed in the wilderness. This milkshake was my salvation, not only because it was a treat but because I got to see my husband's glorious face for a few minutes. It was also nice to know that Chris was checking up on me. If I died of boredom, at least he would find my body while it was still warm.

Knowing he was coming home each afternoon kept me grounded. It allowed me to break up the day in smaller increments, BC and AC—Before Chris and After Chris. As the hours passed, I lay in my lounge chair staring up at the cloudless sky, grateful for the vitamin D the sun provided.

One morning I thought back to the time I'd come home from summer camp to find that my father had spent the whole day indoors. Rachel was with me, and as I ushered her to my bedroom, embarrassed by his unkempt hair and the coffee stains on his shirt, I mumbled, "It's his day off; he's not feeling well."

I was physically bound to my home because of bed rest, but my father was also a prisoner, unable to break free of the constraints of his own demons. Just who and what those demons were, I was still trying to figure out. Yosh's death was the catalyst that catapulted my father into depression, but there had to be something else, some deeper reason, which I had yet to uncover.

I powered on my laptop, wishing I could google the answer. Instead, for no good reason at all, I began looking up statistics about miscarriages and high-risk pregnancies. I knew this wasn't healthy, that I'd only become more anxious, but I was searching for something tangible among the numbers and percentages, knowing that if I couldn't solve the riddle of the past, perhaps I could see the future.

At 4:00 p.m., the end of the day for most but smack in the middle of his, Chris pulled into the driveway. He opened the deck gate, pants smudged with shop dust, sweat dripping from his brow, cell phone propped to his ear, saying, "If the blades are bent, it means you probably hit something." He rolled his eyes. The man on the other end of the phone was so loud that the robin in the lilac tree fluttered her wings. "I can't fix it over the phone, but I can have someone come pick it up tomorrow." The voice got louder. The robin flew out of her nest.

Chris was still holding the milkshake. I willed him to step closer. I wanted to lick the condensation dripping down the sides of the cup. I reached my hand out, but he only said, "I'm sorry, we're backlogged and won't be able to get the mower to you before the end of next week."

He turned to me as he hung up the phone. "The girl at the ice-cream store has it waiting for me now. I just run in and pay, and there it is on the counter. Saves me an extra few minutes." He leaned against the railing, still holding the milkshake.

"Great." I reached out my hand for the milkshake, salivating, but it was not forthcoming.

"Work has been hell," he said, fixing his eyes on Mohonk Mountain House in the distance.

"Sorry it's been so hard for you." *Give me milkshake! Baby want milkshake!*

"You would not believe some of these customers."

I nodded in sympathy, but he wasn't looking in my direction. *MILKSHAKE!*

"We're ridiculously busy."

"Um, can I have the milkshake?" *Don't make me cut you.*

"Oh, here, sorry." He handed it to me. Our fingers touched. I reached out with my other hand, taking his wrist to pull him closer.

"Why don't you sit for a minute?"

"I can't. I've got a million fires to put out."

I let go.

Studying his face, I could see faint lines crisscrossing his forehead like battle scars. I leaned toward him to kiss him goodbye, but his dried, cracked lips landed on my forehead. I began referring to this as the old-lady kiss because it is so devoid of passion that I assumed this is the way a man kisses his grandmother. Only a year before, I'd been dreaming of castles and llama farms. Chris left and Satchie Red stuck her nose between the deck ballasts to get one last whiff of his scent.

The next day we headed to the lab for a three-hour gestational diabetes test. This is a condition that can pop up during pregnancy but goes away shortly after delivery. The stakes were high because I had failed the first test, which meant there was a good possibility that I did have gestational diabetes. Now they needed to find out for sure. I was as nervous walking into that lab as I had been walking into my high school SATs. The lab could not accommodate my bed-resting body, so I pushed three chairs together in the waiting room and slid my legs between the armrests to lie down. I had hoped Chris would keep me company—it would've been a good time to reconnect—but he dropped me off and left to grab a bite to eat and run errands. I knew he was taking time off from the shop during peak mowing season. I also knew that Chris deserved time to eat a sandwich in peace, but I had the opposite problem. My days were too quiet, and I needed human contact.

The results came back that I had failed the second test, too. This meant no more milkshakes. Sugar is bad for pregnant women with diabetes. Not only that, but all carbs were out. I was down to cheese, cashews, and a minimum intake of baby carrots. We'd also be removing all the sharp objects in the house because there was a small chance I might become violent without my daily fix.

I had planned to recline in the car when we arrived at the drugstore to pick up the prescription for the blood glucose meter, but the lure was too great. There were real live people here. I could stroll the aisles, compliment someone's shoes, ask for information on the side effects of Tylenol, browse the nail polish, and pick out a new shade of lip gloss.

When the pharmacist handed me the blood glucose meter, I eyed it like it was a carburetor. What the hell was I supposed to do with this thing? Chris and the pharmacist had no idea either, so we decided to test it out. I hated needles, and now I'd have to stab myself five times a day. It must've been karmic punishment for a previous life's crime. I closed my eyes and jabbed my finger. Then I rubbed my blood on the strip. Nothing. I did this three more times before I began to feel woozy. It hurt to stand. I sprawled my body out on the bench in the waiting area, frustrated and annoyed, while Chris and the pharmacist read and reread the directions.

Feeling sorry for myself that the only way I was allowed to leave the house was if there were body fluids involved, or some other invasive procedure, it took me a while to notice that Chris was using his own blood to get the meter to work. The man was stabbing himself for my benefit—it was the first time anyone had voluntarily bled for me. I couldn't say if it was the hormones or the creeping feelings of depression I was trying to ignore, but I blinked back tears. This was beautiful; this was love. In all honesty, I couldn't be 100 percent sure I'd do the same for him.

He came over and showed me how it was done, stabbing himself two more times until I got it. It reminded me how much I loved him. We hardly talked anymore, and our romantic life was so stale it had grown mold spores. He was overwhelmed and stressed, and I was beginning to worry that he didn't truly see me anymore, or even remember who we were as a couple. But then he would come through, and I couldn't imagine surviving any of this without him. He was my anchor.

When we got home, I told Chris to add the carb-filled Cheerios to the dog bowl with my mother's meatballs. So far it seemed that the only one benefiting from this situation was Satchie Red.

With no more deliveries from the milkshake fairy, I no longer saw Chris until well after dark. But deep down in my soul, there was a tiny seductress clawing her way out over the clamor of rattling prenatal vitamins, blood-sucking machines, and endless Netflix movies. Practically tethered to a bed, with a swelling belly and pain in my nether regions, I had fight left in me yet. I reached under my pillow and opened my brand-new tube of tutti-frutti lip gloss.

13 | The Art of Conversation

Week 24

"I think we should hang a mosquito net above our bed." It was time to rev up the romance. We were going on six weeks of bed rest and my space needed sex appeal. I thought netting would add a certain je ne sais quoi, leaving the door open for a little role playing. I felt around under the sofa bed and pulled out my tiara. "I'm a princess with chiffon scarves and a canopy bed," I continued.

"You are divine and I will do anything your tender heart desires. Let me find the ladder and get to work right now, my fair, witty, brilliant lover."

Okay, that's how the conversation went in my head before Chris came home from work.

"Can we drill a hole in the ceiling?" I said as he planted an old-lady kiss on my forehead later that evening.

"What?"

"I want to put up a mosquito net. It's sexy."

Blank stare.

"Please?"

"I just finished paying off that basement beam. We are not putting holes in the ceiling."

It was true; we'd learned our lesson regarding the fragility of our little farmhouse only months before we were married. Chris had been puttering around downstairs, hiding from the wedding planning, when he happened to glance up at the rafters in the ceiling. To this day he's not sure what made him do it; perhaps he registered a subtle noise, or maybe it was instinct, or maybe God just tapped him on the shoulder and said, "Heads up, dude, this is gonna cost you a lot of money." But he couldn't figure out exactly what he was looking at. Whatever it was though, it was rusting. After further investigation, he discovered that there was a CAR FRAME holding up the house. A rotting car frame. It is a total game changer when you're going about your business in your basement and you see the skeleton of a 1954 Chevy pickup above your head. You have to wonder, *How is it I never noticed a car frame in my basement ceiling until this very day?*

We can only surmise that Chris's grandfather, whom he called Pop, had felt that the car frame would support the house for a few decades. And so it had. But now that time was up, and we spent our first twelve thousand dollars as a couple on one single beam to ensure the house stayed standing, especially since, according to Chris, we were never ever leaving. So with that in mind, it was decided that I did not really need a pink frilly mosquito net.

This was a minor setback, but I wasn't giving up on romance so easily. I lay in bed thinking about fate, about how the entire universe conspires just so two people can meet and fall in love in a supermarket. I wondered what my father must have been like when he first met my mother. There was a picture of him hanging in the hallway by the steps in our house that I stopped to look at from time to time as I was leaving for school. He was maybe midtwenties, leaning on a hot rod like he was James Dean, tall and slender, with brooding blue eyes and dark hair that flipped into a small pompadour with neatly trimmed sideburns. The story goes that a mutual friend had slipped him my mother's phone number on a napkin, but my father didn't think much of it. It was only weeks later, when he dialed my mother thinking she was someone else he had previously met, that he made a date with her. But it was a happy accident, because less than a year later, as they strolled down Thirty-Fourth Street on their way to a car show at Madison Square Garden, my father asked, "Hey, Hochie, want to get married?" Hochie was a shortened version of my mother's difficult-to-pronounce maiden name. Hochie said yes, and shortly after, my father presented her with a ring his mother had picked out.

I have no recollection of my father ever holding my mother's hand or sitting close to her on the sofa, but when I was really young, he'd come home from work and fall into her arms, sharing a long, passionate kiss that caused me to run away in genuine disgust. Late in the evenings, I'd overhear him telling her dirty jokes at the kitchen table, and when they reminisced about the past, I could sense the love between them. Maybe I didn't need big nets and fancy scarves after all.

The next afternoon I ripped off my boulder-holder bra, took my allotted two-minute shower, and then pushed, squished, and molded my boobs into a strappy maternity dress. I had flowers sent to Chris's shop and slipped on my stiletto bedroom heels with the black feathers. I could no longer take two steps in them, but they looked damn good in bed. While I waited for Chris to come home, lounging there in my dress and high heels, I came up with a plan.

When he walked through the door with Chinese food, I asked him to break out the Tiffany champagne glasses we had gotten for our wedding and fill them with seltzer and a spritz of juice.

"Nice shoes," he said. I patted the mattress and gave him an inviting look as he handed me a glass. "I get so bogged down with work. It's a relief to come home." He pulled back the sheets and collapsed next to me.

"We have to celebrate. I'm at week twenty-four. The baby is viable."

"My little family," he said, rubbing my belly and resting his head on my shoulder.

"We have a living room straight out of *That '70s Show*, the house is falling down, you're a ball of stress, and I'm confined to bed, but this child is growing. It's like the baby is sucking the life out of us to feed its own. Oh my God, we have a vampire baby. The baby is going to kill us."

"I don't think that's going to happen." He draped his arm over me.

"There's a real chance our baby will live."

"The baby would have a lot of problems if you were to give birth now."

"True, but every day that I don't give birth brings us one step closer."

"I've been thinking," Chris said softly. "When things calm down, we should plan another trip to Costa Rica."

"If only we could teleport to those hot springs in Arenal."

"Remember the midnight hike through the jungle, and the turtles?" He snuggled closer.

"Life changes so fast," I mused.

"That's how it goes," he said as he rubbed his head lightly against mine. "Those leatherbacks were massive. And their eggs were like dinosaur eggs." His voice was getting sleepy.

"And that water bug!" I shuddered, hiding my head in the nape of his neck.

"It wasn't that bad."

"It was a beast."

After a late-night trek to watch giant leatherback turtles lay their eggs in the sand, we headed back to our boutique hotel in Tamarindo, a seaside town on the Pacific coast of Costa Rica. Just as we got into bed, I spied a water bug the size of my hand crawling up into the corner of the room. I jumped, my high-pitched squeal frightening even the sleeping howler monkeys in the trees outside.

"That was one of the first times you got to see me in full panic mode."

"Well, I always had an inkling it was just under the surface."
He nudged me.

I had demanded the water bug's immediate extermination,
but by the time I shoved Chris out of bed and explained that
he absolutely must annihilate the creature, it was gone.

After that I tried to sleep, making a deal with myself that
I would open my eyes one last time for a quick look around.
Directly above my head was a spotted green gecko scurrying
across the ceiling.

"The gecko pushed me over the edge," I added.

"I thought it was cute." Chris slurped his tongue in and out
like a lizard, leaning in to lick my face.

Upon seeing the gecko, I'd catapulted out of bed and ran
in circles around the small hotel room until I felt something
hard crunch beneath my bare foot. It was a crab.

"You know, I'd never flattened a crustacean before," I said.

"Well, luckily the guy with the pistol showed up." Chris
grabbed my hand and kissed it.

Moments after I had called the front desk about the zoo in
our room, a short man knocked on the door. He had a gun
and a broom. I hesitated. He didn't speak English, and I spoke
even less Spanish. I explained as best I could that I'd take my
chances with the water bug and the gecko.

The hotel owner came by after the guy with the Glock left
and offered us the suite next door. We packed our suitcases
then stepped outside our hotel room, door locking behind
us. At that exact moment the power for the entire hotel shut
down. I completely lost any semblance of sanity.

"I thought you were going to divorce me as soon as we got
stateside," I said.

"I wasn't planning to wait that long."

It was pitch black, we were in the jungle, we couldn't find
our new room, and I was pretty sure something was slithering

up my leg. I spent the rest of the trip with a bottle of DEET on the nightstand.

"I don't know why we don't use DEET here. I bet it would take care of our wolf spiders," I said.

Chris laughed. It was a sound I hadn't heard in a while, and it felt good. His laughter was contagious, and soon I couldn't catch my breath. It wasn't even that funny. We were just looking for an excuse to be happy. He grabbed my face and turned to kiss me full on the mouth as I slipped off my shoes.

Seduction.

14 | Puttin' Up a Fight

I was seven years old the first time I attempted to run away.

"Pack your bags! We're leaving," my brother had said, standing in the doorway of my room where I was giving my stuffed dog George a spelling test. (George was actually a stuffed cat, but at the time it wasn't up for discussion.)

Though Mark and I fought constantly, I was young enough to still hold a deep admiration for him, and nothing could unite us faster than a perceived parental injustice. I didn't know what they had done to cause such upheaval, but it didn't matter. My big brother was inviting *me* on an adventure. I filled a large garbage bag to the brim with dolls and stuffed animals. Then I grabbed my scarf, wrapping it twice around my face, and put my coat on, zipping it up to my chin. "Ready," I said. My mother barely looked up from the kitchen table as we headed out.

Downstairs in the vestibule, Mark turned to me. "Let's wait here." I stood by my brother's side, breathing into my scarf, ready for his next command.

"I'll spy on them," he said.

"Let's just go." I wanted to blow this popsicle stand, travel the world, cross the street!

"Wait here." He ran upstairs, leaving me sweating in my giant puffy coat. I pictured my father beating him, my mother holding him down. After ten minutes I walked up the steps, and instead of seeing bloody carnage, I saw my brother sitting on the floor next to my father watching a ball game.

"Let's go," I said to Mark in a last-ditch effort to start life anew.

"Maybe tomorrow."

"I have gymnastics tomorrow."

"He shoots! He scores!" my father shouted. His team was winning.

"Why didn't anyone come and get me?"

"Eh, we knew you'd figure it out eventually; you're a smart kid," my father said, uninterested in exploring the details of his children's not-at-all-well-thought-out plot to run away. I grabbed my garbage bag and stomped back to my room. I'd like to say I wised up after that, but this scenario unfolded nearly the same way two more times before I realized that a) my brother's threats to run away were just threats, and b) my parents already knew that.

I peered over my pregnant belly and down at my legs, which seemed so far away. I certainly wasn't *running* anywhere now. I used to have rock-hard thighs and shapely calves, but these, along with so many other lithe body parts, had vanished. Fare-well, quadriceps! If I had known you'd be leaving so soon, I probably wouldn't have spent so much time doing spin classes and drop squats. The thought of putting on my cross-trainers and running out the door with a hastily packed garbage bag full of belongings—though these days I'd opt for Kate Spade purses instead of stuffed animals—made me laugh to myself. I wasn't fooling anyone. I could barely walk, let alone sprint to freedom. I had been on bed rest less than two months and my mobility had declined drastically. Every time I hoisted myself into a standing position and took a step, whether it was to pee or to answer the door, one hip would freeze up and I'd be paralyzed while ligaments and bones struggled to correct themselves.

I could only bear witness to the slow, relentless disintegra-tion of my body. At every turn something new failed me: first my uterus, then my cervix, my blood sugar, my joints, the list went on. I had a stockpile of vitamins, pills, glucose tests, and medications lined up by my bedside. I sympathized with elderly people who lived inside flesh and bones that couldn't keep time with their soaring spirits. I knew now what it meant to be in pain every single moment of the day and how it could change someone's entire personality. I tried to appreciate each little joint, artery, and nerve ending, saying silent prayers that nothing else would fail and that this baby inside me would somehow thrive against all odds.

The only way to battle this rapid decline was to become proactive about my care before I crumbled like a pillar of salt. My OB-GYN practice had a policy that you needed to rotate through every doctor in the office because whoever was on call the day you went into labor was the one who would deliver your baby. They wanted to make sure you had already met the person who was about to pull a live human out of your body. But each doctor had offered different and often conflicting advice . . . take vitamins, don't take vitamins; get up, lie down; a little exercise is okay, don't move at all. Besides that, I was uncomfortable having a different doctor checking out my lady parts every other week. I had met all the doctors at least once, and now for my own sanity, I needed some consistency. I told them going forward, I would only schedule appointments with one doctor.

After much obsessing, a couple of lists, and a conversation with Watson, I chose the doctor in the practice who told the best jokes. He had just the right balance of *we're going to do everything we can for you* and *for the love of God, do not panic.* Also, from what I had heard, he was a damned good surgeon, and if it came to that, it was this guy's face I wanted to see in the OR.

At the next visit, the nurse handed me a white paper sheet as she ushered us into the exam room. "Undress and drape this across your lap," she said, turning away.

"What happened to those pink paper robes?"

"Budget cuts." She shrugged.

We waited so long that Chris peeked his head into the hall to see if we had been forgotten. When the doctor walked in, he clasped the tips of my fingers in a way that said, "*Enchanté, madame,*" and then bowed, sweeping his arm out and flicking his wrist up. He stopped just short of kissing my hand. This was his standard greeting.

"Any questions, concerns, problems?" Dr. Enchanté began.

My instinct was to retort with witty banter, but this was not an Upper West Side bar, and my husband was sitting *right there,* so I composed myself and launched in. "God's wrath is raining down upon me."

"Well that's probably not good for the baby."

"My hips feel like they have been freeze-blasted by aliens."

"Yes, well, extraterrestrials are irksome. But I think there is a more logical explanation." He tilted his head and raised his eyebrows to see if it was okay to proceed. I nodded. "You have hip dysplasia," he said.

I was almost disappointed that there was a clinical name for it. Dr. Enchanté suggested I hire a massage therapist to improve circulation and relieve the pain. I knew there was a reason I liked this guy. When else would I be able to justify having a massage therapist come to my house every single week for months? Plus, he thought my insurance might actually cover it.

Thus began a great battle of wills between me and a faceless monopoly. As soon as we got home, I called the insurance company: "Your wait time is now eighteen years, four months, three weeks, one day, two hours, and six minutes. Please hold, and enjoy the mind-numbing music. If you choose to hang up, we will call you back in three years." By the time a representative answered the phone, I had to restrain myself from yelling, "I NEED A MASSAGE!!!"

The insurance company's eight-thousand-page manual suggested they would pay for alternative care, but they initially refused. Didn't matter; I had nowhere to go. I kept these people on the phone for so long, by the time I was done with them, not only did they agree to pay for a bunch of massages, but they promised to buy me a new car and offered me a trip to Hawaii. Not really. But close.

As I was wrapping up my negotiations with the insurance company, I saw Chris heading to the far end of the field with a shovel and then clearing the grass off a huge mound. When he didn't come back in the house, I made my way to the deck to see what he was up to. He was probably getting ready to bury me, but if that were the case, I preferred to be under the lilac tree.

"What's the shovel for?" I called out.

"Woodchucks. They're taking over the garden."

"So you're building them a new home?"

"Gotta get rid of them." He walked closer to the deck so we could talk. "I was hoping you wouldn't see, but I'm going to smoke them out of the garden and bury them in the woodchuck mound."

"The what?"

"I could shoot them if you prefer."

"What mound? With what gun?" The man comes home in the middle of the day and is suddenly obsessed with shooting woodchucks and burying them in a so-called woodchuck mound? So many questions.

"My father's .22. He used to sit on the deck and shoot the woodchucks, and then he'd bury them in that big mound over there." He nodded in the direction of what was apparently a woodchuck pyre, smiling at the thought of his father's antics. "It was a sight to see, Aileen. Him against the woodchucks. All-out war."

"And you're the new general? Why would you kill them? Have a heart."

"Don't judge me."

"No, have a heart!"

"It's a warzone out here. The woodchucks are eating the kale, the chipmunks are digging holes in the flower beds, and the snakes are living in the foundation of the barn. The mice have moved into my father's old Wheel Horse tractor. There's a wasp nest under the motion light. I'm losing control." He was bordering on hysterical. Well, as hysterical as my stoic husband could get.

"I mean Havahart traps." Communication was so hard. "Catch and release. It's like jail for small animals. We have one in the barn." The woodchucks and I could be under house arrest together.

"Hmm." He paused before continuing, and I could see the cogs turning. "Okay. I'll set one now. We'll see what happens. In the meantime I'm getting the mound ready for plan B. I've been thinking, I want to scatter my father's ashes there. It would be poetic. He and his enemies coming together at last."

Was this guy serious? I think he was serious. The man was going to shoot an animal and then bury it in the backyard WITH HIS FATHER. This just doesn't happen in Brooklyn. I'd never seen Chris shoot a gun, and though I knew we had them, I had hoped he would never use them. When I'd moved in, his father's guns were still scattered about the house, the .22 in the corner, ripe for the woodchuck taking. But as soon as I got pregnant, I made Chris buy a lockbox and store them away.

Chris set up the Havahart trap in the backyard and then went back to shoveling. I wondered if this was about the woodchucks or his father. Maybe this was how his family grieves—years later, by shooting small animals. He was finally ready to honor his father by taking on Mission: Annihilate Woodchuck.

We had mourned our losses so differently. After the hospital called to tell him that his father had died, Chris was calm and collected. I display more anguish merging onto a two-lane highway on a good day. When his father's ashes were ready to be picked up a few days later, Chris's mother and stepfather came upstate to provide moral support. They stopped by the funeral home and then went straight out to dinner, inviting me along. A little over two months into our relationship, it had felt a bit premature, but circumstances being what they were, I didn't have time to overthink it. Of course I would join them, but before we ate, didn't there first need to be a bout of mandatory lamenting, soul-crushing regret, endlessly replaying all the things left unsaid? There wasn't even a plan to sue the doctors for malpractice. And most alarming, I could not sense one solitary ounce of unnecessary guilt.

The night my father passed, my mother, brother, and I threw ourselves on the floor in dramatic agony. After leaving AmeriCorps and moving back into my mother's house, I spent mornings focused on freelancing, but by noon I was sitting on the floor in the dark, narrow hallway, knees up to my chin, my face ravaged by tears. Even if Chris didn't talk about his feelings, I knew deep down he must still be steeped in grief, and I wanted to be there for him. I just needed to find a way to do that *and* protect the woodchucks.

With Chris still digging around the mound, I saw something in the trap moving. Usually it took days to catch an animal.

"Chris, you caught something!" I shouted. Maybe now he would stop channeling his Austrian farmer persona, and I could go back to staring at the walls and worrying about health insurance.

He picked up the trap, and there inside was a baby woodchuck. "I'm taking him for a ride," he said.

"You let that baby go right now."

"What? I thought we agreed."

"I'm not joking. That baby needs its mama."

"He's destroying my kale." Chris held the Havahart trap in one hand, looking up at the deck and arguing with me.

My hormones were raging. My breasts ached just thinking about that helpless little woodchuck whom my husband might or might not release into the wild miles away.

"You're not taking that baby away from its mama."

While Chris stood there pleading his case, the little brown woodchuck ran in circles, clawing at the metal cage. I could see him trying to squeeze his body through a tiny gap. I kept Chris talking, negotiating, buying time. The woodchuck found an escape hatch and ran.

"Run, baby woodchuck, run for your life. Your mama's waiting," I shouted. Chris turned around to see what I was talking about, watching in awe as the tiny Houdini ran back toward the garden.

"I can't believe that just happened," he said.

"I love you! Don't be mad. I needed to save the baby. We always save the babies."

"I'm going back to work." He put down the shovel and got back into his truck.

"Do you want me to take the beer stein with your father's ashes off the mantle so you can sprinkle it on the mound?" I called out, but he didn't hear me over the rev of his engine.

A few days later the doorbell rang its shrill song and Satchie Red's reign of terror commenced. I shuffled my way over to answer it. It was near impossible to take even the smallest steps. Outside, a woman with long brown dreadlocks stood marveling at the view of the ridge. Satchie Red was barking, strings of drool reaching the floor. My dog's wide eyes said, "I will eat this woman; she will be my dinner."

"Just walk past her. This is the only thrill she's had in days," I explained to my new massage therapist. As Becca made her way into my kitchen, Satchie Red's demeanor changed and she began rubbing her head against Becca's bare legs. This bohemian angel with radiant ivory skin was dressed in a floral frock and strappy flats. She smelled divine, like lavender, or flowers, not quite perfume, more of an essence. Sometimes it's nice to be a dog; while Satchie Red rubbed all over Becca, I was resigned to appreciating the scent from a socially acceptable distance. I hobbled over to the counter to find a paper towel for Becca to wipe the drool off her leg.

Becca did her best to tend to me, but Satchie Red demanded equal attention. She jumped up on the massage table, straddled my legs, and waited her turn with Becca's magic hands. We coerced her off the table, and just as I began to relax, I heard a lapping sound. She was eating the massage cream. Becca, to her credit, did her best to ignore Satchie Red, but these were not the working conditions she had in mind.

Along with the hip dysplasia, I had sciatica. The pain radiated down the side of my leg, and if I didn't know better, I'd almost believe someone had cut me open in my sleep, inserted a sharp knife, and then sewn me back up. No mere human was going to tame the Monsters and their wily ways, but Becca did perform miracles. Toward the end of our first session, she told me to lie on my side. She placed her hands under my belly and then lifted ever so slightly. In an instant she had taken away my burden, relieving the pain and pressure, and in doing so, she gave me one beautiful, fleeting moment of freedom. Time stopped as she both physically and spiritually lightened my load. I handed her my hopes, my future, my sweet, tender dreams of being a mother, just long enough to remember who I once was. With this simple gesture, she had accomplished more than anyone else had been able to.

Then wham! The baby punched Becca hard, jolting me and surprising her. "You've got a little fighter in there," she said.

15 | Blame It on the Cossacks

Week 26

I opened Salman Rushdie's *Midnight's Children*, held it above my head, but lost interest before I made it to the second paragraph, my arms aching. There was a stack of unopened books sitting by my bed.

I had often fantasized about a forced hiatus where I could catch up on the classics and while away the hours. But the dark secret about this fantasy is that you only end up on a forced hiatus if something bad is happening to you. I was locked away, the world spinning along without me. I looked over at the unread pile of books and then up to the wood-paneled ceiling. This is what the inside of my father's coffin must look like. Then, because I had frightened myself with that thought, I reached for the books and arranged them in the bed around me as if they were my talismans.

It was the children's librarian at the Kings Highway Library who had first sparked my love of words. She had pin-straight brown hair parted in the middle and thick round black eyeglasses. Her plaid A-line skirts reached mid-calf and made a soft swishing sound as she floated through the stacks of books. For the life of me I can't remember her name. She was kind but serious, and she loved Ludwig Bemelmans's *Madeline.* Because of her, my career path was set by the time I was nine. I wanted to be a librarian just like whatever her name was. But my father had other ideas. "You're going to be a truck driver," he said. I was a dainty girl who looked very much like Shirley Temple, and

I spent my afternoons in my mother's closet trotting around in high heels and applying her lipstick. "Wipe that stuff off your face and come over here." I stood before him. "Take off those shoes before you kill yourself and put up your dukes!"

I complied, scrunching up my face with my best mean look as I raised my fists.

"Throw with your right, block with your left. Loosen your fingers." He was not going to leave his little girl too soft and tender for this tough world. But after we went a few rounds, he pulled me onto his lap on his Archie Bunker chair and let me paint his fingernails.

I held my pregnant belly and rolled to my right side, shielding my eyes from the light streaming through the window. I looked up at the ceiling again: my wooden coffin. Before his burial my mother, brother, and I had to identify my father's body at the funeral home. Jews have closed coffins so this was the only chance we had to make sure it was Richard Weintraub being buried that day.

As we lined up in front of the casket, the funeral director asked if we were ready. I gave the smallest nod and swallowed hard. He opened the top half of the lid first, and I looked at my father. He didn't look so bad. I put my lips to his forehead. He was cold. I hadn't expected him to be so cold. The director opened the bottom half and stepped away to give us privacy. "Where are his shoes?" I asked. "You don't need shoes in heaven; God pulls you up by your feet," my mother answered.

We had brought a recording of Liza Minelli's rendition of "Cabaret," and played it while my mother sang the words. It was my father's personal theme song, and he did make a happy corpse, as the lyrics suggested.

When there was nothing more to do or say, I walked into the sitting room and leaned against a wall, wrapping my arms around myself. A blur of faces offered condolences, and I nodded my thank-yous, watching the scene unfold as if I were a spectator instead of one of the lead characters in the main event. My father's closest friend, Paulie, stood in front of me and said, "Richard was the most brilliant man I've ever met. He was the only person I knew who could convince both his children that each was his favorite." Paulie was right. Both Mark and I still claim the title. But that was the first time anyone had referred to my father in the past tense, and it broke me.

I rolled over to my right side and began tracing my hand along the knots in the wall paneling, half singing, half humming the lyrics to "Cabaret." At the end of the song I said out loud to my father, "Well, old chum, I hope you're celebrating."

I reached for the remote and clicked on the television to channel surf the morning shows. Every day of bed rest was a conscious decision. This could be a day that I spent looking at the wall, or a day when I felt part of the greater world. Determined to keep my head above the surface, I focused my attention on the morning show.

And so I began a secret affair with a new man. His name was Produce Pete. He was a robust older gentleman with a familiar New York accent. Not my usual idea of sexy, but he was talking about picking the ripest, freshest goods on the stand. This man was the real deal, hearkening back to the days when my mother and I would go to small fruit stands in Brooklyn to buy our vegetables. He was talking about strawberries, and I was hooked. It wasn't lost on me that I had somehow developed a pattern of falling for men who knew a thing or two about produce.

I grabbed my laptop and looked online, as I often did, obsessively memorizing fetal milestones. I did some quick calculations and figured out that by the time Produce Pete was showcasing radishes, my baby would hopefully weigh just over a pound and his or her brain development would begin to speed up. I thought ahead, wondering if I could maintain this pregnancy until Pete began his segments on nightshades—eggplant, tomatoes, peppers. I'd be a full seven months pregnant, and my baby might have a healthy shot at life. I tried to hold on to the idea that apple season, when my baby was due, was just around the corner.

I dozed off, and when I awoke I was crampy and anxious. I'd always lived my life with a low hum of anxiety buzzing in the background, but the stress of being on bed rest had amped it up, and it was manifesting in my dreams.

Though practically doctor-prescribed, I was starting to dread my daytime disco naps. What should have been a guilty plea-sure, a mark in the pro-bed-rest column, became the catalyst for a whole new list of worries. I didn't even have to be fully asleep for the nightmares to begin. Every time I closed my eyes, they were there, waiting: My baby was gone. Stolen. Dead.

After waking up from another of these episodes, I called Watson.

"I'm having nightmares. I'm in this bar, and the birthing center is across the street . . ."

"You need concrete," he interrupted.

"Like for mixing?"

"You live in the middle of nowhere. That's why you feel like crap. Come home. For the love of God, get out of there, woman! It's not too late!" Watson had been telling me to "come home" since the day I had moved to Saugerties.

"There's always so much blood in my dreams."

"Arterial spray or spillage?" I heard his chair squeak as he leaned back.

"Spray. No, spillage. Not helping."

"Why don't you work on *The Ten-Second Seduction* again? Given the circumstances, I don't think your husband will be jealous," he continued.

"Do I sound seductive to you? How am I supposed to be sexy? I have Monsters growing in my uterus."

"Monsters are sexy. Remember Dracula? Not Bela Lugosi, I'm talking 1979 Frank Langella, when he was in his prime."

"Who?"

"Everyone forgets he was one of the best Draculas."

"What is your point here?"

"Use this experience for your book. Seductresses get pregnant all the time. I mean, if they're good at what they do. You know, the seducing part."

"Okay, fine, let's talk about the book. I'm getting stuck writing about Yogi Man," I said.

"Have you noticed that people who do yoga are the most stressed-out people?"

"True, Yogi Man was a tormented soul. So I think the lesson should be . . . what should it be?"

"Don't do yoga."

"No. More along the lines of we're all struggling."

"And doing yoga makes it worse."

"Well, it brings it to the surface. And then I can explore whether or not that's helpful. You know, repression does have its place. Look at my husband's family. They're experts at stuffing it all down. Sometimes we need to make a conscious effort not to suffer so much."

"Right. Everything better now? 'Cause I got a meeting," he said.

I got the feeling Watson was getting tired of hearing about my cervix and all the problems that went along with it. I got this feeling mostly because every time I spoke to him, he said, "Have this baby already. I'm tired of hearing about your cervix and all the problems that go with it."

Maybe he was right. Maybe what I needed was concrete. Here in the country, with my friends and family far away, I felt alone. In Brooklyn I had a support system. Unfortunately, the main player in that support system was dead.

On Tuesday evenings, while I was still working in the city, I'd head over to my parents' house for dinner. One night as we were finishing dessert, I began telling my dad about a coworker who'd betrayed my trust. It was one of my first lessons in office politics. My father went over to the kitchen counter where he kept his Absolut and poured me a vodka on the rocks. "Drink this, then we'll talk."

He and I headed to the living room and sat on the floor watching old *M*A*S*H* reruns as I told him the sordid tale. He lay on his left side, propped up on his elbow, and then he opened an AARP magazine in front of him, using it as a place mat for his ashtray and his second vodka of the evening. Without turning his head from the television, he flipped his right wrist up, palm open, and said, "Who the fuck cares?" He handed me his lit Newport. I inhaled deeply, allowing the menthol to seep into my lungs.

Those four little words, "who the fuck cares," became a cathartic mantra I've since used to deal with more than a few of life's hurdles. My father had given me some useful tools to get along in this world. Vodka, a cigarette, and a one-line catchphrase turned out to be a handy arsenal.

Unfortunately, if there ever was a time that vodka and a cigarette just *weren't* the answer, this was it. I couldn't brush off bed rest or even my nightmares with a firm "who the fuck cares?" This time I really did fucking care. I cared about this baby and I cared about my relationship with Chris, which meant I also cared about fourteen-inch replacement blades and Toro Wheel Horse 8-25 air filters. Suddenly there was an endless tide of things to care about.

"Where are you now with your 'who the fuck cares,' Dad?" I asked aloud. I was angry. Angry because for all his work trying to make me tough, he'd forgotten to tell me what to do after the vodka was gone and I'd smoked the last cigarette. At some point we all have to confront our issues or they consume us . . . like they had consumed him. Oh. Right. So maybe he didn't forget to tell me what to do; maybe he just didn't know. I swung my body around to lie next to Satchie Red. "Well I finally have a big-girl glitch." Satchie Red stood up, shook her wrinkly chops, and settled a few inches away.

I dialed Chris at the shop. "I need a Ouija board."

"You have the wrong number."

"I'm serious."

"Me too."

"Maybe therapy would help," I said.

"For me or you?"

I had been going to a therapist on and off since I was twelve years old. It was like a bat mitzvah present for neurotics. You're twelve, you're a woman, here's your very own therapist, enjoy.

But now, the logistics of speaking to a therapist while on bed rest seemed insurmountable. Even if I could do phone sessions, I'd have to find one who understood my circumstances and then try to develop a rapport. By the time a new therapist was caught up on all my baggage, my baby would be applying for a driver's permit.

Chris came home that evening holding a small metal object in his hand. "This three-quarter-inch tire bolt has been giving me problems for the last hour."

"Looks intimidating," I said from the sofa bed. Satchie Red was now standing on my legs like I wasn't even there, wagging her tail at Chris's arrival.

"How was your day?" He threw the bolt on the table.

"Not so great." I gave Satchie Red a shove, and she jumped off the sofa bed.

"I had this one customer today, called six times to find out when his tractor would be ready."

"I'm having nightmares, during the day," I said. "How come we don't call them daymares?"

"You always have nightmares. A few months ago you stood on the bed screaming and pointing at the ceiling. I had another customer who wanted to return a tire he bought a year ago."

"I did not stand on the bed. Why didn't you tell me?"

"I'm used to it. Ever since you insisted I fold laundry at 3:00 a.m. two weeks after we were married."

"Yeah, that time I wasn't sleeping."

"So anyway, I tell the guy, you can't return something from a year ago. Didn't even have a receipt. Who does that?"

"In this dream I'm in a bar, I've just given birth, and there is all this blood. I'm still attached to the IV."

"It's just a bad dream. You'll be fine. Then I had a customer who bought a tractor a month ago. Tells me he wants to return it. I go outside to take a look at it, and the guy bent up the whole left side, must've hit a tree. Now he doesn't want it anymore."

"I'm not fine, and you're not listening!"

Chris was out in the world every day making money and pursuing his dreams. I knew it was hard for him, but he wasn't trapped. He was building his life, while mine was on hold.

"I'm sorry. I'm doing the best I can. I'm trying to tell you something, too. What do you want me to do about your nightmares?"

"I don't want you to do anything."

"Can I make you more comfortable? Do you want another pillow? What if we go out for dinner?"

"We can't go out for dinner. I can't get out of bed. I just want you to sit here. And listen. I want you to listen."

"Okay. Let's talk about your dream." He got into bed next to me. I looked at the side of his face, the way his ear, cauliflowered from a jiu-jitsu injury, puffed out at the tip.

"I don't want to talk about it anymore," I said.

"Just tell me." He put a hand on my thigh.

I considered giving him the cold shoulder for a few more minutes, but I was eager to talk. "Like I said, I'm in a bar, and the neon sign in the window is blinking on and off, and I'm trying to shield the baby's eyes." As I spoke, I rested my head on his arm and I could feel him soften into me. It felt so good to have his full attention. "Why was I in a bar with a newborn? What kind of mother am I going to be?"

I heard a gurgle. I looked up and saw his head back, mouth opened. He was asleep, the sound coming from his throat, deep and guttural, not unlike that of a small brush hog.

"Chris, are you listening?"

"Yes, yes," he said, roused. Seconds later his head dropped to his chin. Well, at least one of us had no problem sleeping. I lay there, thinking back to the winter morning I told him I was pregnant. In the short span between then and now, something unrecognizable had grown between us like a sharp and stubborn vine. I was alone. Here, with my child growing inside me and my husband sleeping next to me, I ached for a connection with at least one of them. They were both so close, but I couldn't reach them.

I looked around the room. The house, too, felt like an acquaintance that kept me at arm's length. Chris's grandfather's cowbells hung on a hook; his father's wood-carved owl perched on a shelf. My memories here were topical, recent. I had no history, no portraits on the wall. I could no longer access the small studio space with my belongings that Chris had set up for me across the property. The only items we could claim as *ours* were a bookshelf, a dresser, and a new mattress. I grabbed a pillow to my chest and hugged it tight.

I gave up trying to talk to Chris that night, wishing I could pick up the phone and call Rachel. We would spend entire afternoons deconstructing our dreams, consulting books and searching for hidden symbolism. And then one day she said we shouldn't talk about these things anymore; she was becoming more religious, and it didn't feel right to discuss symbolism outside of Judaism. Missing Rachel, I picked up the phone and dialed my mother. I told her about my dream. After a long discussion, we mutually decided it would be best to blame it on the Cossacks. The Cossacks are a thing in our family, and my mother has a propensity for fitting them into conversations that have absolutely nothing to do with Cossacks or war or Poland.

"Why don't I come for a visit?" she said abruptly.

"Sure, after I safeguard my house against Cossacks we'll plan something," I said.

"Okay."

"Listen, Ma, before you go, have you heard anything about Rachel?"

"No, I haven't. Do you want me to ask around?"

"I guess not."

Finding a confidante who would listen to me was proving difficult. Much easier was recruiting support for things like groceries and other errands. I was anxious for obvious reasons, but there was so much more to it than saying, "I'm feeling these emotions because I might lose my baby." It was more like, if I lose my baby, then what? Where do I find the strength to move on? And what about my marriage? It was under so much strain already; I knew in my gut that we would fall apart. I had given up my career, my freedom, and my ability to move to keep this baby alive; how would those things ever matter again if my baby didn't survive? This wasn't about feeling sorry for myself. This was about figuring out who I was and what I was capable of handling.

I was disappointed in my doctor for not mentioning how psychologically strenuous bed rest would be. It's a fact of life that people miscarry. But like bed rest itself, it doesn't seem to hold a lot of weight out there in the world. How would I recover?

That night, tossing around in bed, it was more of the same bad dream. I woke with a start at 4:00 a.m., consumed by the irrational fear that someone was trying to break into our house. Not long after my father quit his job in the garment district, I became preoccupied with home invasions. I awaited the day a masked man would burst through our door, slice open my parents' throats, and sell me on the black market. I have no idea how I came up with this elaborate plot. Perhaps it was that one time after watching the news with Dan Rather, when my mother turned to me and said, "Creeps would love that curly hair of yours," or maybe it was when my father had jokingly whispered in my ear that Dracula roamed the streets of Brooklyn sucking the blood from little children. Whatever the reason, I had some deep-rooted fears.

One rainy night, when I was about six years old, lying in bed, eyes wide open, I had worked myself up into such a frenzy that I jumped up and ran down the hallway to our living room in my fuzzy footed pajamas, convinced that I was being chased by something I couldn't see. My mother picked me up and carried me back to my room. She tucked me under the heavy comforter and in a firm voice said, "Stay in bed," before turning to leave. Deep inside my closet, with its chipping plaster walls, there was definitely not a secret door that led to a witch's coven, but try telling that to an overtired child. I lasted all of five seconds before running after her, clinging to her satin chemise, begging her not to leave me. As she was prying my little fists from her nightgown, I heard my father's voice: "I'm warning you, Aileen."

He stood up slowly. Lithe he was not. The floor groaned beneath his feet as if the giant from "Jack and the Beanstalk" had just stirred. *Fe Fi Fo Fum.* "Get to bed!" he shouted. I put my hands on my hips and widened my stance: "No!" He scooped me up, carrying me to my room. I kicked him in the gut and pounded his chest, trying to bite him. He dropped me on the bed and left, but I could not be alone in that dark place. I ran after him. He stopped and turned, and I swear the whole house rattled with fury. He picked me up by my elbows, pulled me so close to his face that I could smell the remnants of the anchovy pizza he'd had for dinner, carried me down our steep flight of steps, opened the door, and put me on the stoop. The lock clicked behind me. I pounded on the door and screamed until my pajamas were soaked through with rain and the sweat of fear. Someone let me back in, hours, minutes, seconds, later. Most likely my mother, and probably not so much out of love but because I might wake the neighborhood.

My father and I never discussed the incident, but from that night on, he tucked me into bed and then sat on the floor of my room watching the small black-and-white television set, and I learned more about Larry Bird and the Boston Celtics than any other first-grader in Brooklyn. He stayed with me almost every night until I was about twelve, and after that I slept with the overhead light on until the day I moved in with Chris. Somehow my father had managed to be both my dragon and my knight rolled into one.

Now, I turned to face my husband in the dark, watching his chest rise and fall. He was my knight now, and he would protect me, but here I was once again worrying about home invasions and child snatchers, both real and invented. I squinted to see Chris's features, the outline of his full lips, the curve of his chin, the stubble of his beard. I wondered if my new knight had his own dragon inside of him. I couldn't imagine it. I threw my leg over his strong, lean body and gazed past him until I drifted off to sleep.

I woke up exhausted and called Jackie to invite her over for breakfast.

"I don't eat breakfast," she said. "But I'll come."

Satchie Red alerted me to Jackie's arrival. She came in, put a bag of pastries on the sofa next to me, and then plopped her small frame down on the pink-and-blue-striped chair. Tying her red hair back into a bun, she launched into a list of physical ailments: arthritis, phlebitis, diverticulitis. I couldn't keep up.

"You think you have it bad? Getting old bites. Just wait." She meant it to be humorous, but I didn't smile. "What a sour puss on your face. Tell me, honey, what's up? I'm going to help you." Just the invitation I'd been waiting for!

"I have this recurring dream. I'm balancing my big post-partum body on this red leather stool in a bar, and a zombie dressed as a hospital orderly comes barreling toward me. He looks around frantically and then grabs my baby. I refuse to let go. But he's yanking my child out of my arms. I don't know if the orderly got my baby. Jackie, I have to find out if he got my baby."

Jackie widened her green eyes, placed both of her pale sun-spotted hands on the arms of the chair, leaned in, and said in her harsh smoker's voice, "Listen, honey, the first time a woman has a baby she's scared shitless, whether or not she's on bed rest. And now these doctors are telling you something's wrong. Of course you're having nightmares. All this newfangled technology with the testing and the pictures, I don't know if it's so good. What has it done for you? Nothing. It's giving you so much stress. Bastard doctors." She sat back in the chair, throwing both her hands up.

I let the truth of Jackie's words settle.

"This is temporary, a small blip. Soon you'll be able to put it behind you," she continued.

"I hope so," I mumbled.

"This is not a problem. A problem is something you can fix. You can't fix this, so it's not your problem."

"Interesting logic."

"You want to hear problems, let me tell you what my grandson was caught doing." She shifted on her hip. "This grandson of mine, a problem. My phlebitis. That's another problem."

"What happened with your grandson?"

She leaned in close and whispered, "Drugs." And then louder, "I'll kill 'im. Look, you have to do something else. Try knitting." She stood up to go. "I'm coming back. Tomorrow. I'll bring more pastries."

"Thanks, but I can't eat pastries. Gestational diabetes."

"Okay, so you'll watch me eat them. Maybe you'll have a bite."

After that I began talking to Jackie almost daily. She was always home when I called, she never tired of hearing about my cervix, and not once did she mention Cossacks. As soon as she picked up the phone, I could hear the strike of a match and the clink of an ashtray. She settled in for the same conversation we'd been having for weeks.

"Honey, honey, I keep telling you . . ." She paused to take a long, deep puff. I waited with bated breath for her to exhale. "It will all work out. There are big changes coming for you. I feel it in my bones."

16 | The Hex Upon Us

Week 27

Jackie told me that it would all work out, but she didn't tell me that the road to it all working out would be riddled with land mines. Every time I tried to redirect my thoughts, they would turn back and explode into fragmented feelings of inadequacy. *I deserve this pain. I will never be good enough to be a mother. My marriage will fail.* Was this what it was like for my father, lying on his own couch, self-deprecating thoughts spiraling around in his head as he stared at the ceiling? Did he forgive himself for his mistakes? Did he regret them? Did he regret me?

Richard Weintraub had not been a kind man. He was short-tempered and solitary. His immediate response to all requests was a resounding "no." On the weekends, when we still had a car and I was too young to take public transportation, I'd ask him to drive me to my friends' houses. If I somehow convinced him, he'd mutter under his breath the whole ride, making sure I'd think twice next time. In seventh grade, as I trudged home from school in a blizzard, the wind whipping around me, snow and ice pummeling my face, I expected him to meet me halfway to lighten my load, guide me, but he only appeared when I finally reached our corner. "Where were you?" I asked.

"You did it. You're fine," he responded. Yes, it was true, but I had wanted him, needed him, to be there by my side.

And yet he had been there. At fifteen, after I was snubbed by my latest boyfriend, my father sat across from me at the kitchen table as I wiped away tears of unrequited love.

"Why are you with this guy?"

"I like him."

"You like that he makes you cry? You can do better," he said, grabbing a tissue from a nearby box and tossing it to me.

"But what if—"

"No what-ifs. What does this guy do for you?" he cut me off. I stood up to go back to my room and digest his words. "And don't put out. It won't get you anywhere," he called after me. It was good, honest advice. He had asked the right questions, and pointed out the obvious. He was teaching me to think for myself. But I still longed for tenderness. Perhaps that was why, when the rabbi had asked what I saw in Chris, I answered that it was his kindness. My father had never gone out of his way to be kind to anyone, including himself. That was where I needed to be different. If I could step back and look objectively at the girl on the bed, I could see that my body and my soul were in the midst of great trauma. The nightmares were my subconscious expelling the toxic negativity that had built up inside me. If I could stop judging myself so harshly, if I could be just a little softer and patient, maybe I could find a way to quell my own doubt and self-loathing instead of letting it consume me the way my father's had consumed him.

The day before he died, he was practicing his own version of self-care. He bought a Greyhound ticket and spent the day in Atlantic City, gambling and strolling the boardwalk. He was happy there, dining at a buffet and bellying up to the bar. What better way to go out than winning a few rounds of blackjack and coming home with a pocket full of cash, the sound of the ocean still echoing in his ears?

I was in no condition to board a Greyhound, but I did have a laptop, so I switched it on and pulled up the season's hottest dresses, belts, bags, and strappy sandals. I couldn't fit into them and had nowhere to go to show off these lovely accoutrements, but I had deep faith that if you purchase a to-die-for item, the universe will bless you with an event to wear it to. I set my sights on a red Kate Spade clutch that was marked "Final Sale." Wrists and fingers swell, feet elongate, and baubles do not hang right with a pregnant belly, but an elegant clutch goes with all of life's seasons.

With a nod to my dad, I dropped that little purse into my virtual shopping cart, reached for my credit card, and entered my payment information with wide-eyed anticipation. And then, there it was, flashing in red on the screen: DENIED. I tried another card. That, too, had the same sad outcome.

I felt a familiar dread creep up my spine and remembered the fight to end all fights that my parents had when I was in the third grade.

"I can't take it anymore, Gail." His eyes were glued to the green velvet wallpaper in the living room.

"You had no right to take that money. Who do you think you are?" Her pitch was high and strained, and I could see her red-rimmed hazel eyes holding back tears.

"Who do I think *I* am? Who are *you*?" He turned toward her.

"You left us with nothing," my mother said, steeling herself. On the tortoise-shell lamp table beside her, a subtle shimmer caught my eye. It was her wedding ring. I had witnessed many fights, but not once had I seen that thick gold band separated from her person.

She stomped away. For a wisp of a woman, she had a grand exit.

"Mommy, wait. What happened?" I raced after her as my father let the pages of the *Daily News* scatter to the floor while searching for his cigarettes on the shelf beneath the TV.

"We're broke."

"I have bills, Gail. Do you understand that?" he yelled across rooms.

"How am I supposed to buy groceries if we have no money?" she stormed back at him.

I wasn't sure what was going on, only that my father had long since given up looking for a new job.

Here on my sofa bed, waiting for that intrusive memory to recede, I scanned the wood paneling of the sun-soaked room to see if I could find any new Rorschach shapes; today there was a wolf. But if I turned my head sideways, it sort of took the shape of a chicken. I rolled my neck around and looked back at the computer: DENIED. This was how both my parents must have felt in their own way.

Growing up in a house where money was a contentious issue, I became an avid saver and planner. I thought that marrying Chris would mean financial stability. He didn't balk at my feast-or-famine freelance lifestyle, and he wasn't worried about money, so I took that to mean he had plenty of it.

I had never missed a bill payment before, and I couldn't understand how this had slipped by. Chris had been trying to hold us above water, and I hadn't even noticed that we were drowning. The shop brought in more bills than we had expected, and they were piling up at a rapid pace, but in my malaise, I mistakenly assumed it was under control.

And now not only did we have to pay the bills we already had, but we were counting on there being another human in the house soon. My belly started twitching. The baby was hiccupping.

I dialed Watson.

"Babies need lots of stuff. Did you know that?" We no longer wasted time with hellos.

"Yes, yes I did. My wife and I have been known to occasionally provide for our own children." Watson had a boy and a girl.

"We can't pay for it. Do you understand what I'm saying?" I rubbed my belly to soothe the baby.

"No." I heard the clicking of his keyboard.

"My mother had a friend whose baby used to sleep in a dresser drawer instead of a crib. Is that still socially acceptable?"

"Hey, guess what? You're making plans for your baby. That's new. Plans that will have Child Protective Services at your door, but hey, it's a start."

"I'm not ready to be a mother."

"Stop. Just stop. You're fine."

"I wish everyone would stop telling me I'm fine. I'm really not fine."

"That's okay, too. Nobody's really fine. Everybody is dealing with their own stuff."

"So you're saying I'm just like everybody else?"

"Yes. You are absolutely ordinary."

"I don't really understand our friendship."

Feeling better despite his usual brutal candor, I hung up and clicked on the television just in time to catch Produce Pete's spiel about snap peas. It was the end of June, and snap peas meant I had thirteen weeks of bed rest to go.

Shopping was out. I needed a new plan. If I wanted to buy something, I'd have to put it on my baby registry, which I still wasn't mentally fit to tackle. Though I *could* wrap my mind around the idea of a bed-rest registry. I was pretty sure I could pass off that Kate Spade clutch as a diaper bag. With a little ingenuity, I could fit one nappy, a small tube of lanolin, and a binky in there.

When Chris came home, I asked him to lay out all the bills on the bed. He disappeared momentarily, returning with a huge plastic bin meant for Christmas ornaments. Now it was filled with legal envelopes in various states of distress. Some were ripped open, others only partially torn into as if subjected to a scornful and rapid glance, and some were altogether untouched. He dumped them on the duvet. There had to be almost a hundred of them. I thought it was a joke.

It was not a joke.

Chris and I were in slippery territory, and I was beginning to see striking similarities between him and my father that I hadn't picked up on previously. They both kept their worries to themselves, sometimes to their own detriment, and because of this, there was a lot of miscommunication. My dad and Chris were both quiet people—loners. They didn't go out with friends or have anyone to hash out their feelings with before coming home. But Chris worked hard; he had a plan for our future. By the time I was old enough to know what was going on, my father had given up on a better life, but I now understood that, like Chris, he'd once had dreams, too, even if they were as far-fetched as becoming a private investigator.

"Forget it. Just throw them in the garbage. No way we're able to pay all of these," I said. He began to collect the envelopes and put them back in the big storage box. "What are the odds they'll throw us in the clink? They wouldn't put a bed-resting broad in prison, would they? You head back to Brazil and take up jiu-jitsu again. What's their extradition policy anyway?"

"I didn't think you'd want to know about this," he said.

I appreciated that on some level, but I also felt duped. I had thought we were in this together. "Well now we need to deal." I sighed. "Give me that box."

Devising a financial plan was the last thing I wanted to think about, but deep down I knew even a bedridden woman, perhaps especially a bedridden woman, should always be aware of her money situation. There had to be ways to tighten the proverbial belt at the same time my own belly was expanding. I quickly got to work.

Some things were no-brainers. First I changed our cable package, since mostly I was watching Netflix anyway. Next up was renegotiating our cell phone service. I wasn't using any minutes, so I cut that, too. Finally I ordered a book—from the library—about financial planning. I learned how to consolidate credit card debt and transfer balances to zero-interest cards.

I also started thinking about long-term financial planning. I knew a baby was going to put a dent in our budget, so I needed to figure out where the extra dough was coming from, lest I come up short at the drugstore on a late-night baby wipe mission. I couldn't yet envision our child's lips, its brow, its cute little button nose, but I could start saving for college.

Taking an active role in the family finances gave me a feeling of control when I was losing so much of it in other parts of my life. It was difficult for Chris. He wasn't used to sharing his financials with anyone. During his parents' contentious divorce, there were questionable dealings around money, and so he'd learned to hold his own assets close and to trust no one, but if he gave me the opportunity, I could show him how to stretch a dollar. I might not have been bringing in serious bank, but I wasn't spending a whole lot either. I was saving money on gasoline, dining out, dry cleaning, entertainment, and of course my former daily coffee fix, not to mention food, since I only really ate baby carrots. I also found that most companies were willing to work out payment plans. Chris never said it, but in his own way he expressed relief that he no longer had to carry the burden alone, like when he'd ask about a bill and find it already paid.

Even with my finagling, we came to the uneasy conclusion that we were going to have to draw against our home equity. I hated doing it, not knowing how or when we would pay it all back. I had seen my own parents on the verge of bankruptcy and could not, would not, relive those days. We hoped that if we held tight, the shop would eventually turn a profit. We'd heard that when you buy a business, you have to wait five years before coming out ahead. Five years? Who has that kind of time?

Luckily, as a real estate agent before buying the lawn and power equipment shop, Chris had gotten a really good deal on a rental property, and we had tenants already living on our farm in the converted barn. He also still had one or two contracts pending with clients waiting for closing dates. He was now juggling three full-time jobs (property manager, agent, and new business owner) along with taking care of his bedridden wife while renovating our bedroom/nursery suite. It suddenly seemed like I had the better end of the deal.

I was counting on our rental income to get us out of our financial hole, but Chris dropped more bad news. One-third of our rental units were vacant. We were bleeding cash, and even worse, the tenants who remained were coming undone.

One night the local sheriff called to inform us that a tenant was swinging a machete around the front yard while yelling obscenities. A few days later we got another call that a tenant was dealing drugs and we could be fined if we didn't do something about it. The world we were trying to create together was crashing and burning, and all I could do was watch it smolder. It felt like there was a hex upon us. Every time I tried to take a deep, cleansing inhalation, the baby would lodge a limb in my rib cage. Even breathing seemed impossible.

But if I could pack up my city life and move to the country, if I could wear non-wicking GORE-TEX through treacherous winter hikes, I could get these apartments rented. This became my new life's mission. Hadn't my father taught me to get back up when life pushed me down? These lessons had not come easy—for me or for him. By the end of seventh grade, my father had gone back to work driving a cab for Busy Bay Bee Car Service in Sheepshead Bay. The play on words was a source of endless amusement for my budding literary brain. He hated driving and his eyes were cloudy from glaucoma, but this was steady work during the recession years.

Every afternoon, I came home from my long, grueling hours at Cunningham Junior High to an empty house, where I waited until 5:00 p.m. to call Rachel when her bus dropped her off from yeshiva. She was my lifeline, my saving grace. The bullies at Cunningham made my life hell, but Rachel was a constant source of comfort and, during those years, my only friend.

The two years I spent at Cunningham, a place of unbridled agony, were the loneliest, most difficult times in my life. It was every kid for herself; alliances made one day, unraveled the next. The boys teased and taunted me about my budding breasts and flat ass, but the girls were downright vicious. Angie Marino was a frizzy-headed brunette with freckles who looked around Spanish class one morning and chose me as her target. She passed me a note with a slew of creative names, some of which I didn't even understand. Beneath this well-thought-out letter was a stick figure scene of her plunging a knife into my heart. The notes became more threatening and detailed, with a warning that she was planning to jump me and that if I were smart I'd crawl into a hole and die. All the good holes were already occupied, so I took my chances with Angie. Also, I wasn't really that smart. Back then there were no policies against bullying, and Cunningham was a place where the weak were devoured. The school was so overcrowded, with at least eight or nine classes of up to thirty kids per grade. No doubt the administration would have been happy to lose a few.

Though Angie didn't live near me, her apartment building was a block from my orthodontist. When my father asked why I kept missing appointments, I was forced to confess.

"Deck her," he said.

"She'll crush me."

"So what?"

"You haven't seen her. She's big."

"Never show fear. A'ight, here's what you do. This girl confronts you, tell her to fuck off. Really loud, like you mean it."

"I'll be dead."

"Tell her, 'FUCK OFF.' If she lays a finger on you, don't run. Stay and fight. Right hook to the jaw, jab with your left. Upper cut under her chin. All else fails, grab her by her hair and go for the eyes. Otherwise she'll keep tormenting you. Just don't be stupid about it." I took that to mean "don't miss."

"Block your face. Those braces are expensive," he continued. "I'll get in trouble."

"With whom? I'm the only one you have to worry about. Someone hits you, hit back harder. Remember," and here he slid his glasses down his nose, peering over them, "never start a fight, but you damn well better finish it. Or don't come home crying to me." I was twelve years old.

A few weeks later I was in Angie's neighborhood and she was sitting on a low brick wall surrounding an apartment building on the corner of Ocean Avenue. I could feel her eyes shooting lasers at me. I had to pass right by her to get to my bus stop across the street, but my sympathetic nervous system was begging me to run in the other direction. I thought about braving oncoming traffic and crossing in the middle of the four-lane avenue instead of heading for the light, but I remembered my father's words. I held my head up high and looked straight ahead. She sniggered and called me an ugly coward. This was it. It was now or never. "Fuck off," I said. Okay, I whispered, but I had said it, and I know she heard it, because she smirked. I didn't wait for a response before picking up my pace to cross the street, pleading with the traffic gods that the light would change before she decided to jump off the wall and slam me to the ground. I looked down the avenue, thankful that my bus was just a half block away.

This would be a better story if she stopped bothering me after that, but life isn't neatly tied together with a bow. She continued to bump me in the hallways and belittle me, but I was less afraid of her now. She'd had an opportunity to take me down and she hadn't.

Now, like then, I had a choice to make: I could lie in my bed, a damsel in distress, allowing waves of hopelessness to wash over me, or I could do something about our financial situation. I would get the apartments rented, hex or no hex. It'd be a lot easier than facing Angie Marino.

17 | Power Equipment + Bed = Sexy

Week 27½

As the calls from prospective renters came in, words I never thought I'd string together came out of my mouth:

Yes, dogs count as pets . . . Oddly enough roosters do, too. Last I checked, sir, wives do indeed count as another person . . . So do children and mothers-in-law. Sorry, no, your mother is not a good reference. I don't know if your grandmother's furniture will fit in the small bedroom. I really can't say how many settings the shower head has, and yes, marijuana smoke is included in the no-smoking policy. Please don't call if you're undecided about whether you even want to move. I'm not your guru. I'm on bed rest, damn it! Can't you people figure out your own lives?!

Each time I spoke to a potential applicant, I felt like I was betraying my father. Every month before paying the rent, he'd look at me and say, "Kabeen, landlords are a rare breed, don't ever forget that." It was a cryptic warning I didn't understand, but it was probably because he loathed handing over his hard-earned cash to someone else. Maybe he felt that he should have been the landlord, and perhaps someone other than two thankless kids should have been beholden to him for shelter.

It took time, but eventually I found tenants. This added to Chris's workload, showing the apartments and fixing them up, and each day I could see another layer of exhaustion take over his already lean body as more pounds fell away. I had wanted to help Chris with the apartments and the business, and though he was grateful, it didn't bring us closer in the way that I had hoped, and it didn't take any pressure off him. Now, on the rare occasion that we had time to talk, it was all business and money, and disagreeing about strategy. It was hard for him to relinquish control; he both wanted and resented the help.

As I was turning in one night, I nudged Chris, who'd again fallen asleep while I was talking, to get washed up and come to bed for real. Instead, he got up to paint and scrape the wallpaper in the nursery. I wondered what he thought about while working into the wee hours of the morning. Did he think about tractors, customers, bills, what kind of father he'd be? Did he think about how hard it was trying to hold it all together? Did he think it was worth it? That I was worth it?

In the morning, on my way to the bathroom, I peeked in to see what he had accomplished in the nursery the night before. By now he must be almost finished. Instead, I could see that because he had been painting with only one small, low light at night, and was exhausted, there were multiple spots along the wall he had missed. It would have to be touched up, maybe even redone. One step forward, two steps back.

Chris called me from work. His office manager had a fight with one of the mechanics and stormed out. The office manager had been there for years, and she knew a lot more than Chris about the day-to-day operations. Chris, God bless his soul, thought that he could take on her workload. There was no conceivable way the man could shoulder any more responsibility. A few days later, Chris's driver cut his hours, saying that he preferred to focus on his music. Chris said, "No problem." He could do that, too.

When he came home that evening, I handed him a book of matches, reminded him where we kept the lighter fluid, and told him that as far as I knew, he'd been home with me all night. He responded with a maniacal laugh and wandered away. For a moment I wondered if he had taken me seriously and had gone to light the shop on fire, but then I heard him rummaging in the pantry for a snack.

That night I heard the cries of scavenging coyotes as they surrounded the house. It sounded like they were climbing up the siding. Once the coyotes found their victim (a neighbor's cat, a stray chicken), they commenced their high-pitched heckle. The sound was so unlike anything I had ever heard, I questioned if I was really hearing it. But Satchie Red, brave, fierce warrior dog that she was, cowered deep in the back of her kennel, moving nary a paw. I knew that I was going to wake the next morning to a bloodbath in my yard—bones, feathers, clumps of fur, bloodstained grass. In Brooklyn if we woke up to such a sight, we'd report it to authorities; here it was normal. When the coyotes slunk back into the darkness, I was left with the familiar stirring of anxiety.

Panic Phase 1: What if I survived and Chris died? The man was so stressed that he could have a heart attack at any moment.

Panic Phase 2: How many ways might Chris die? What if he were driving the diesel and fell asleep at the wheel? What if he died of paint fumes, or starvation?

Panic Phase 3: What would become of me after he died? An anxious pregnant lady trying to run a tractor store from bed and living on a farm overrun by wolf spiders.

It went on like this for a good part of the night, and when Chris rolled over in the morning to old-lady kiss me on the head, I grabbed his face in both my hands. "Don't die."

He raised his right eyebrow. "You're squeezing my face really hard."

"You know how many people cut their hands off with chain saws each year and bleed to death because they can't dial for help?"

"No. Do you?"

"Listen, this is serious." I let go of his face.

"Who had an accident with a chain saw?" He tried to rub the sleep out of his eyes.

"Nobody . . . yet."

"Okay, I'll do my best not to die today. I wouldn't want to mess up your plans."

After Chris left for work, I called Watson.

"Chris is going to die."

"Is he in imminent danger? If not, I have clients in five."

"No, he's fine."

"Are you planning to kill him? I always recommend strychnine. But definitely torture him first."

"He's having a really hard time."

"Yeah, well, we all are."

"He doesn't look so good."

"So tell him to relax."

"Yes, I'm sure he just forgot to do that." I rolled my eyes and explained to Watson everything that was going on. I didn't know how much more Chris could take.

"Why don't you do it?"

"Do what?"

"Manage the shop. You're a control freak. It's perfect."

"Watson, you're brilliant." With his love of horror movies and talk of guts and spillage, Watson was the least likely person I'd thought would get me through bed rest, but he never failed to come up with rational advice, and what's even more surprising is that he continued to answer the phone when I called.

As I lay there in bed petting Satchie Red with my feet, because she never let anyone get close enough to pet her with their hands, I toyed with the idea. I'd be the remote representative of the shop. I could work from home, paying the bills, updating files, writing advertising copy, and placating customers. Chris had been talking about tackling warranty work for weeks now—surely I could do that, whatever *that* was.

We would save money by not immediately hiring a new office manager and I could learn the business. I grabbed a scrap of paper and wrote the equation *Power equipment + bed = sexy?* I drew a diagonal line through it and crumpled the paper. There was no spinning this. *The Ten-Second Seduction* had no place in my current life.

Chris jumped on the idea, bringing home an oversized red binder to get me started. "Before we begin," he said, "I've been meaning to tell you something. I've always had to figure things out on my own. My dad wasn't around a lot. My mother tried, but she worked all the time. So I forget about you sometimes."

"Thanks for sharing that. I feel so much love right now."

"Let me finish. I forget that you're by my side. You have my back. It means a lot."

"Let's see if you feel that way in ten minutes." I reached out for his hand to pull him down next to me on the sofa bed. I knew that these words were hard for him to say, and I appreciated them.

"Let's start by having you warranty the piston on that Z," he said.

"Okay. No problem. Except what the hell are you talking about?"

"Forget that. Write down the code for the axle, and fill in the item number for the fifty-two-inch Toro deck."

"The deck? You have a deck at work? I didn't know that."

"The deck on the tractor. Can you pay attention?"

"That depends. Can you speak English?"

"Maybe we should try sorting through the invoicing system first," he said.

I nodded and feigned interest, but that, too, was mind-boggling. The last owner had left the books in disarray and everything was *fakakt*.

I tried to do the warranty work and learn the invoicing system, but I simply could not process words like *coil, spindle, hydropump, PTO clutch,* and *lift rod.* Though I was kind of inter-ested in hearing more about this *lift rod.*

I stuck with it for two more days, but it was clear that I would have to obtain an intimate knowledge of tractor parts to do this job, and honestly, that just wasn't going to happen. I couldn't concentrate and I began making jokes, which for some rea-son Chris didn't find very funny. Being in bed for so long had drastically shortened my attention span. I could hardly keep up with the story line on *Judge Judy* these days, let alone pay attention to a rundown on small engine repair.

I called my mother to tell her about our financial crisis. She had been through hard times, and she'd have sound advice, I was sure. After listening to me for a few minutes, she said, "I have the perfect solution for you. Just give me a couple of days."

I knew this was no simple fix. She had something up her sleeve. "Don't do anything batty, Ma," I said, but she had already hung up.

18 | The Vanishing Penis and the Reason I Have a Therapy Fund Set Aside for My Unborn Child

Week 28

The doorbell was stuck as usual, and I knew it would take me a solid two minutes to get out of bed to answer it. Satchie Red was running in circles and rolling her head along the ground like she was possessed. When I finally opened the door, though the bell was still ringing, there was only a brown box sitting on the welcome mat. I unstuck the bell, picked up the box, and glanced over at Satchie Red, who predictably had a thin string of drool on each side of her chops, and I imagine that if she could speak, she would say, "This bell is trying to kill us." I stuck my head around the door and saw the Charlie Chaplin UPS guy sitting in his truck. He waved at me with a smile before pulling away.

The mystery box had no return address. After struggling back into bed, I opened it, hoping to find something glamorous. The inner package was wound tight in five layers of bubble wrap and sealed with silver duct tape. It was either incredibly fragile, or explosive. Several minutes into deconstructing the wrapping, alternating between anticipation and frustration, my suspicions grew, and by the time I tore the last piece of tape off the box to reveal a Tupperware covered in industrial-strength tinfoil, the jig was up. I opened the container and found a partially thawed casserole.

My mother had attached a yellow Post-it with the words *noodle kugel* written on it, and beneath that was a stick figure family, one of which had a giant belly and another that was, I think, supposed to be a dog but looked more like a dead rabbit. I put the kugel aside for Chris. Though not the intent, this half-thawed kugel made me feel like a failure. I had failed at keeping my household running, but even more, I had failed at the very essence of womanhood. How was it that I could be so determined and brave—quitting my New York City job, joining AmeriCorps, moving to the country without knowing a single soul—but the one thing that I had been born and bred for—making babies—literally knocked me down? Then I remembered my vow to be kind to myself. I called my mother to thank her for the package. The first words I blurted out were, "I think it's time for you to come for a visit."

My mother turned out to be the one person who showed up, knew what to do, and had the best advice, maybe even better advice than my father might have had. The last few weeks I had noticed a minute shift in my relationship with her. Sure, we were still pushing each other's buttons, but we were talking more, too. How had she become so smart after all these years? Had she spent my long, insufferable youth waiting for me to come around, filled with frustration, feeling that nobody appreciated her? Regardless, she continued to do what she had always considered her job: caring for her family no matter how defiant or selfish we were. This kugel was not just noodles and oil, and it didn't matter that I couldn't eat it; the main ingredient, the only one that truly mattered, was pure, organic love.

The next day she was at my door.

I lowered the volume on the television when I heard the familiar *thump, thump, thump* of my mother schlepping her schlock-store suitcase up the steps. She came in the house melting from the heat and, with one awkward swing, threw her suitcase up on the pink-and-blue-striped chair. Hands on her hips, trying to catch her breath, she turned to Chris, who had picked her up at the bus stop, and said, "Open it." She pointed at the suitcase. He thought it was a joke; I could see from the look on his face that he was in no way prepared to unpack his mother-in-law's delicates. It was only when she insisted between hyperventilating breaths that he coaxed the zipper around its track and then quickly took a step back as if expecting a cobra to jump out. There was not a single item of clothing in this bag. Instead, it was filled with meat. My mother fluttered her lips and collapsed in a chair as though she had just completed the New York City Marathon.

"Ma, I'm a vegetarian."

"Well I don't know what to make you. You don't eat anything."

"That must be an entire cow."

"You do this to torture me." My mother wasn't trying to be overdramatic. One of the biggest ways she showed her love was through food. It really was torture for her that my diet was so limiting and the one thing she could do in times of hardship—cook—wasn't going to help.

But by late afternoon she had moved on from meat to other pressing domestic matters.

"You want I should use bleach on your colors?" she asked as she hefted a huge basket of laundry on her hip.

"We don't have bleach."

"I brought my own."

"You brought your own bleach? From Brooklyn? They let you on the bus with bleach?"

"How do they know? They didn't strip-search me at Port Authority. It's color safe."

I had no words. But it did make me think: *What exactly is color-safe bleach? Is it even bleach at all? How do they get the whiten-*

ing agent out? A dirty pile of laundry had spurred the deepest philosophical musings I'd had in months.

"After this I'll do the floors. I brought something for that, too," she called out as she left the room.

My mother, much like myself, had a love/hate relationship with cleaning. Every Friday night during my childhood, I watched as she violently pushed the monolithic Hoover across the orange shag carpet. Then she would move on to assaulting the plastic covers on our dining room set and couch with Windex. Nowadays people laugh at plastic furniture covers, but I cannot wait for them to be back on trend—that furniture remained unscathed through years of blood and vomit my brother and I had unleashed on it. Once my mother was done assailing the plastic, she would attack the kitchen floor, getting down on her hands and knees, scrubbing every square inch until she could see her reflection in the speckled linoleum. She got out her aggression on that floor, and when she was done, whatever burden she had been holding on to that day had been absorbed by Mr. Clean's no-wax shine.

My brother and I had made her job more challenging by not picking up after ourselves, and our father was even worse, purposely making work for her. Our kitchen table was divided into two halves that could be pulled apart to make it bigger, and every evening after dinner my mother slid a knife in the crack to clean out the crumbs. It was a mystery how so many crumbs got stuck in that one little space until, one day, I came upon my father eating a ham sandwich, which was totally verboten, and caught him *pushing* the crumbs into the divider. "I like to drive your mother nuts," he said. With two hormonal adolescents and a husband who went out of his way to piss her off, it's no wonder we had the cleanest house in Brooklyn.

By the next morning of my mother's visit, my little farmhouse was sparkling. I headed to the shower, and as I was waiting for the water to warm up, I noticed piles of wet laundry neatly folded and placed in Ziploc bags sitting on the bathroom sink. It was possible that my mother was single-handedly responsible for countless baby seals who had met their demise choking on plastic ocean waste. No matter the explanation, it would never make sense and it would never change, so I didn't ask.

Even though she was an environmental terrorist, by the time her visit came to a close, I was beginning to see how patient and kind my mother truly was. I was almost tempted to ask her to stay longer, but I knew our time together had a statute of limitations. I appreciated her attention to detail and found her idiosyncrasies a welcome distraction, whereas I used to find them unbearable, but for the sake of our relationship (and the planet) I thought it might be wise to hire a housekeeper.

Although well aware of our worsening financial situation, Chris and I figured out a way to have someone come in twice a month. We were so deep in the hole that another few bucks wouldn't make much of a difference, and my mother, feeling it would take the burden away from her, offered to chip in. I searched the local paper and found someone who seemed like a good match.

Josephine, a short, middle-age woman, came shuffling through the door, her hand placed on her fleshy lower back as though she were pushing herself up the short flight of steps. She walked into the kitchen and greeted me with a warm smile. I wasn't sure how well she could clean, but her rate was more than reasonable, and when she was done listing her ailments as though they were things to be gossiped about, and relaying the details of her daughter's boyfriend who was going to school for small engine repair, she looked around and laughed. "You cleaned before I got here."

"No! Well . . . we didn't want you to think we were slobs."

"I don't do laundry or windows. If you're okay with that, I can come back in a few days."

With my mother no longer there to distract me, the familiar feeling of sadness began to seep back in, but now that I knew Josephine would be coming around, I had something to look forward to; I was guaranteed a full day of company twice a month.

I spent the rest of that day watching the clock, waiting for Chris to pick me up for our appointment with Dr. Specialist. We were going to finally find out the sex of the baby. As the hours ticked by, I gazed out the window overlooking the lush green mountains, observing our hummingbirds.

The phone rang, and I scrambled to answer it, hoping that whoever was on the other end would be my salvation. It was a telemarketer. Here, I thought, was an excellent opportunity to make new friends. These people had no place else to be; it was their entire job description to talk to me. They also had good timing, calling right in the middle of the day, which I now referred to as "the endless hours." It began at 1:30 p.m., when the upright world was deep into their work, the sun was at its peak, and there was nothing but reruns on television. It ended at about 4:00 p.m. when the afternoon talk shows came on and I could at least pretend I was experiencing the world in real time.

On the other end of the phone was Joyce from the *New York Times*. I started off harmlessly enough, asking her what state she was calling from and what the weather was like. Then I moved on, asking her if she liked her job, whether this was her career or a stepping-stone. She was happy to chat. Poor Joyce, people were always hanging up on her; no one wanted to get the first month free with a year's subscription. I had a feeling Joyce would appreciate being asked how her day was going, what her kids were up to, and if she had any summer plans. Not long after I hung up with her, the local fire department called asking for money, and I explained that I had an incompetent cervix and money was tight, but since I had them on the phone, did they have some sort of sticker I could put on my window to let rescuers know I was inside on bed rest if there was a fire?

When a debt collector called to harangue us, I knew I had hit the jackpot. His name was Jeff and he was calling all the way from India! I'd never been to India. I was dying to hear all about it.

Chris came home just as Jeff and I were finishing our conversation about his grandson's upcoming graduation.

"Who was that?" Chris asked as he leaned in to kiss my forehead.

I frowned. "It was Jeff. Something about your credit rating. I'm not sure, but do you think we can send his grandson a gift? You know, something small."

"What?"

"He can't be at his grandson's graduation. He's in India. How about a weed whacker?"

"We have to go. We're going to be late," Chris said, not at all interested in his credit rating or Jeff.

We arrived at Dr. Specialist's office and waited our turn with all the other high-risk women. Unlike the OB-GYN's, this waiting room had a much more intense energy; no one likes going to specialists.

The exam always started out the same way. Because of the Monsters, I was the lucky recipient of both a Doppler and a transvaginal sonogram. The tech squirted cold gel on my belly and then rolled the Doppler around, showing me the Monster Fibroids just as excitedly as she was showing me the arms and legs of the baby. Next she measured all the inhabitants of my uterus. I could see the baby's head pressing up against the Monsters like they were trying to suck his brains out, and the biggest Monster was jammed up against my cervix.

"Do you want to find out the sex now?" the tech asked.

Before I knew about the Monsters, at my very first sonogram, eleven weeks along, Sherry from Dr. Enchanté's office had unofficially told me she thought I was having a boy. She didn't want to say for sure because it was so early, but the lady had been doing her job for quite some time, so I figured she had mastered the identification of boys and girls in utero. I hadn't told Chris what she had said because I wanted to wait until it was official. Now I had an opportunity to find out for certain. I nodded, but Chris held up his hand in protest. "Wait. I'm not sure about this," he said.

I turned to the right, and there the technician stood, trans-vaginal ultrasound wand held high in front of her, all gelled up with a condom on the end. I gave her a look that implied this might take a moment. She sat down in her tech chair, still holding her magic wand upright.

"What?" I said, more a challenge than a question.

"I'm not sure I want to know yet. I'm not ready to get attached," Chris replied.

I hadn't considered his perspective. This was a big difference between the two of us. I needed to face life head-on, armed with as much information as possible. Chris liked to take the scenic route, see what unfolded naturally. I could kind of see his point. If we knew the sex of the baby, the next step would be to choose a name. Once we did that, it would be a real live human being to us. Right now it was less a baby and more an idea that represented our future, a grainy picture we could kind of see if we squinted. Maybe Chris felt it would be easier to get over the loss of a baby if we never truly knew much about him or her. But I was already attached to whatever was growing inside me—well, except for the Monsters; they could leave at any time.

"I need to know," I said.

"Let's think about this," he repeated.

In general I think a lot quicker than Chris. He takes a painfully long time to make decisions, and it downright slays me. His brows knit together, his lips purse, and you can almost see the cogs in his brain turning as he mulls over the facts. I knew I had to work on meeting him in the middle, slowing down, and pondering his point of view. But not today.

"Let's make a compromise. You leave the room, and the technician can tell me. I need to know who's in there. I have to know who I'm fighting for."

"Okay, I'll stay." He nodded once, taking his seat.

The technician worked her magic wand as we waited with bated breath. "Well, it looks like you're having a girl," she said with a huge smile.

"No, I'm not," I said.

Chris sat there unfazed. You can't argue with a pregnant woman about her fetus and win.

"Well, I can't be 100 percent sure, but I'm usually right, and I think it's a girl," the technician said.

It's not that I didn't want a girl. I truly would have been happy with any type of living, breathing baby. I simply didn't believe her. I told the tech what Sherry the sonographer had said weeks earlier, thinking that if she'd told me it was a girl and the tech told me it was a boy, I could see that. But a fetus can't have a penis and then not have a penis. Penises, in my experience, do not just go away, not even when you stop answering their phone calls and tell them that, no, you do not want to have dinner with them.

The tech, not knowing what else to say, called Dr. Specialist in for his three-minute celebrity appearance. I was beginning to gain insight into the whole specialist modus operandi. Even though the specialists are the ones with the fancy degrees, it is their techs who do most of the work. The doctor, who must carry an egg timer in his pocket, spends exactly 180 seconds with you, telling you all the things the technician already told you but wasn't supposed to, and then you write a check for eight thousand dollars that your insurance company promises to cover but doesn't.

Dr. Specialist said he also thought the baby was a girl. He admitted that it was hard to tell, and there was a small possibility that the baby's leg was hiding the penis. There's a magic trick if I've ever seen one. Was there some sort of penis pocket stuck to the baby's leg? Where could the penis be?

Because I was insistent, and maybe because I came across as slightly irrational, Dr. Specialist agreed that we wouldn't call it now; we'd check again in two weeks when I came in for my next appointment. I glanced over at Chris, but he had his poker face on. He had gotten his way, after all. With me refusing to believe Dr. Specialist, we had shed only confusion and a hint of absurdity on the situation. As everybody left the room and I got dressed, I looked at my belly and whispered, "You're a boy. I know you are."

19 | Going in Reverse

Week 28½

Early the next morning, my mother called with a new level of urgency in her voice. The Great Annual Mealy Moth Invasion had begun. Like me and my wolf spiders, my mother was plagued with moths and spent a good part of her time methodically plotting their annihilation. She had packed up the entire edible contents of her kitchen—spice rack, peanuts, even canned goods—and jammed them into her refrigerator. You practically had to wear body armor to get to the cheese bin lest an avalanche of lentils, Frosted Flakes, and couscous overcome you.

After much trial and error, my mother had concluded that the best way to exterminate the mealy moths was by weaponizing a Swiffer Wet Jet. With the grace of a trained assassin, she would grab her Swiffer, spin it upside down, and tiptoe over to her victim. Then, with brutal force and stone-cold precision, she would push the dripping mop onto the ceiling to kill the moth, smooshing it with patented Wet Jet technology.

"Mom, I miss you." I had interrupted her account of her double life as a moth slayer/Jewish mother.

"I can't come visit right now. I've just pulled my whole house apart. Don't make me feel guilty."

"I'm lonely in my marriage, Ma. He barely ever comes home."

"What makes you think I have such good advice? My marriage wasn't so great."

"Well, what did you learn from it?"

"I have three boxes of opened matzah meal. I can't even figure that out."

"Ma, focus."

"Okay, well, your father was just like Chris in many ways," she said.

"What? The man hardly worked."

"That wasn't always the case. You just don't remember. When we were first married, he'd never take a day off. Once, I sprained my ankle and needed him to come pick me up from night classes at the college. As he was helping me into the car, he told me that he had to work the next day. Didn't matter that I had two little ones at home."

"Dad hated work. Why wouldn't he take off?"

"I think he was afraid he'd lose his momentum. Maybe he figured if he stopped working, he'd have a hard time going back."

"Well, he was right."

"Trust me, if I had figured all this out back then, the problem would have been addressed somehow."

"So you think Chris is afraid he'll lose his momentum?"

"What do I know? I'm just saying, there may be something else driving Chris that you haven't figured out yet."

"This conversation has raised a lot more questions than it's answered."

"So go find the answers. But don't be surprised if it takes you thirty years of marriage. I have to go deal with my moths."

She made loud kissing sounds before she hung up, and I was left wondering if there was something deeper driving Chris to succeed. Though, according to my mother, I wouldn't figure out the answer for another twenty-nine years.

I heard someone at the door yelling, "It's Josephine, don't get up!"

My new housekeeper appeared before me, huffing from the four steps she had just ascended into our kitchen, with Satchie Red's nose firmly planted in her crotch. The house was still clean from my mother's previous visit, but this was when Josephine was available to start, so I asked her to do the baseboards and other deep cleaning.

Josephine's hair was a platinum poof freshly curled with giant rollers, her eyeliner a perfectly drawn cat eye. "She's pregnant. My daughter's pregnant. Do you believe that? Eighteen years old." She threw her hands up. "I'll start in the bedrooms," she said, ranting to herself.

It was an unexpected greeting from somebody I hardly knew, but her motherly tone of exasperation was both familiar and comforting.

"Do you want me to do the family room next or the kitchen?" Josephine called from the far end of the house fifteen minutes later. How had she cleaned the bedrooms so quickly? I wanted to hear more about her daughter's unexpected pregnancy, so I asked her to spend some time in the family room. It felt funny lying in bed while someone worked around me. I didn't want her to think I was watching her every move, but I also didn't want to act like she wasn't there. It was an unnecessary concern, because Josephine launched into how she was too old to take care of a baby and listed her issues with her daughter's boyfriend.

As she spoke I made some observations about her cleaning methods. She mopped, but with no cleaner. She couldn't reach overhead because of back pain, so the ceiling fans and the top two shelves of the bookcase were left dusty. She didn't bend, so the baseboards suffered, and though she did vacuum, it wasn't her forte and the pushing-and-pulling action made for uncomfortable moans and groans. I couldn't see much of the floor from the bed, or below my colossal belly when I got up to go to the bathroom, so it didn't bother me too much.

I found her to be great company, and her animated stories were worth her reasonable fee.

Josephine went on about her daughter's pregnancy, and I could feel an unexpected jealousy rising from the pit of my stomach. I didn't want to be eighteen and pregnant; I just wanted to have a young body that could support a full-term, healthy gestation. But then, there were people who thought that my position was enviable, too.

"You're so lucky, I wish *I* could stay in bed all day." This usually came from older women who had forgotten what it was like to be pregnant, or how to act in basic social situations. I had been bombarded with opinions and advice, like the helpful, "Rest now! You'll be up all night once that baby comes." One relative was offended by the amount of water I was drinking. I was thirsty all the time, and though I told her my body knew what it needed and I'd be okay, her response was, "I never drank that much water while I was pregnant. You're going to float away." She didn't know the half of it. I had to relieve myself so often that if I could have harnessed my pee into sustainable energy, I'd have been able to reverse climate change.

Shirley, a distant relative, began calling me every day because she was lonely and I was available. It was mutually beneficial until I began to notice a pattern: every conversation revolved around a baby tragedy.

"Did you get tested for Tay-Sachs? I knew a girl about thirty years ago who had a Tay-Sachs baby. Terrible disease," she said.

"I think I've been tested for that. I'm not sure."

"Well, another girl I knew from my knitting klatch, her granddaughter was born with I forget what it's called. But no good." This was the worst possible thing to say to someone with anxiety because I couldn't even google whatever it was she was talking about; I could just stress out over the endless possibilities.

I didn't want to know about difficult births, NICU babies, or infants with little chance of survival. I wasn't close enough to the finish line to wrap my mind around birthing, never mind all the things that could possibly go wrong afterward. I didn't have a baby yet, and I might never have a baby. With so many tragic stories, it's a wonder anyone is ever born at all. And if indeed one was lucky enough to make it through the birth canal alive, growing up to adulthood seemed near impossible.

I stopped listening to everyone's horror stories and unhelpful advice. Bad things happen every single day, but if I was going to obsess over other people's misfortune, I'd never have the strength to confront my own.

Josephine moved on to the kitchen, mumbling to herself about the cost of diapers. Continuing to sit with my jealousy, I placed a yoga block under my sacrum to take the pressure off my cervix. The general idea was to be inverted as much as possible but not entirely upside down; this was no easy feat. There was so much tension in my lower extremities. I was physically trying to hold this baby inside me with every muscle in my body. As I worked on relaxing my pelvis and quadriceps, I allowed the yoga block to support my weight. I envisioned my baby growing strong, clenched fists, a little jiu-jitsu fighter. I could see the viscous fluid surrounding the baby, enveloping it in layers of protection. I felt raw and exposed, but this child was safe in my womb. I pictured the umbilical cord not only supplying life but flowing between us.

The phone rang.

Trying not to disrupt this elusive state of Zen, I felt around the bed for the handset, peaceful and Buddha-like at first and then, with the unrelenting ring demanding attention, much more frantically. The machine picked up and the generic voice came on stating there was no one available to take the call—as if! Of course I was available! Where else would I be? I finally found the phone buried beneath the sheets.

"I have a little problem with the Pathfinder," Chris said.

"Little?" If it were little, he wouldn't have called.

"Well, it doesn't go backward anymore."

"Umm, why do you need to go backward?"

"You know, reverse, it doesn't go in reverse. I was towing tractors and I blew something. Maybe part of the transmission."

"You were what?"

"I was in a hurry and the diesel was down; I figured it would be fine."

"Can it be fixed?"

"Well, it's still drivable. Like you said, who needs to go backward? Also, it would cost a couple grand."

I fell off my yoga block.

After we hung up, I hugged my knees to my belly. Deep breath in, deep breath out. I tried to regain the energetic connection with the baby, but it was no use. The moment had passed. I wanted to cry. Every day I fought the vicious beast of depression. I was winning, but it lurked just beneath the surface, and it would take only the smallest ripple to rise up and burst through the fragile veneer.

Chris called again toward evening. "I'm going to be late," he started off innocently enough, but I could feel the bad news coming.

"Okay. Where are you?"

"The post office. I can't get out of the parking lot. I've been maneuvering for a while, but I can't get the right angle to make the exit."

"I can't even begin to process this." It was damn funny picturing my husband circling the tiny parking lot, notorious for its inaccessibility even with normal, reversible vehicles. "Take your time and God be with you."

"I'm an atheist."

"Well maybe it's time to reconsider, 'cause I don't know how else you're going to get home tonight."

Chris finally walked through the door—three days later. Well, it could've been, but he got lucky and was home in just about an hour. The parking lot cleared out enough for him to make an exit without divine intervention. Of course he could have called someone for a ride, but that wasn't in his nature. He was literally driving in circles, unwilling to ask for help.

I considered offering to let him drive my Honda for a while, if he promised not to tow tractors. There was a problem, though. I didn't really want him to take my car. What if there was an emergency? What if the phone lines were down, if there was a storm, if my road had to be evacuated because of an unexpected bear migration? Besides, my car was my last vestige of freedom. As long as I had wheels, I could still Thelma-and-Louise it the hell out of here. I wasn't sure I wanted to share my symbolic lifeline with him.

Reluctantly, I took the keys from my night table, about to hand them over, and then I paused, keychain suspended, dangling by my thumb and forefinger in the air. Chris looked at me, reaching up for them in slow motion as though we were both making a deal with the devil. We had become so delicate, trying to hold on to whatever was ours, not wanting to give up anything, not even to each other.

20 | The Muck and the Mire

Week 29

Chris came home from work before the sun set. I had high hopes when I heard the screen door slam. Perhaps we'd have dinner together. As he planted his usual kiss on my forehead, he told me he was going to mow the overgrown lawn. I could have asked him not to; I could have suggested he sit beside me and talk, but the truth is, I wanted the lawn mowed more. There were so many chores that had been left unattended. The outside of the house was unkempt and the grounds had gone wild. I longed for some semblance of order. I heard him rummaging through the cabinets, opening a bag of chips, eating cashews, biting into an apple.

"You're not taking care of yourself. I'm sorry I can't prepare meals, but you're eating like a closet mouse."

"I know."

"What's going on with the Pathfinder?"

"Still at the mechanic."

The mechanic had called multiple times to confirm that he had fixed it and we could now safely reverse once again. He wanted to know when we were picking it up, but with only one driver in the family at the moment, we had the logistical problem of getting both cars home. I began hiding under the blankets when the phone rang, afraid he could see me with his X-ray phone vision. He left so many messages that Satchie Red had taken to barking whenever she heard his voice.

Chris had gone over to pick up the Pathfinder, but with no way to get two cars home without—God forbid—asking someone to go with him to drive one of them back, he left the Honda there. This leaving one car for another had been going on for days. The mechanic didn't care that I was on bed rest. In the most recent message, he threatened to tow.

"Don't worry," Chris said. "Eventually I'll bring over the big diesel from the shop, drive the Pathfinder up on the flatbed, chain it down, and take it home. Problem solved."

"Yeah, nothing could go wrong with that plan."

The next sound I heard was the sweet purr of a small engine; music to my ears as I recalled the scent of freshly cut grass. I enjoyed the hum for a good ten minutes, until a high-pitched whine, an excruciating sentiment of frustration and failure, broke my reverie, and then the engine cut. Moments later the whining resumed, and I recognized it as the whir of wheels spinning in futility. I moved to the lounger on the deck to bear witness. Chris was down at the field's edge near a thick line of tall spruce trees that had been planted too close together long ago when Pop had the idea of starting a Christmas tree farm.

I watched as Chris placed his hands on the rear of the big red zero-turn and began pushing, his feet sliding behind him. This was a huge tractor. Its deck alone was seventy inches across, and I was impressed with myself for knowing what that meant. Only, this wasn't exactly our mower. It belonged to the shop, and it had to be back in the morning to be loaned out to one of the big kahuna landscapers.

Chris alternated between turning the ignition and pushing from behind, refusing to acknowledge defeat. He looked up to the sky as though pleading with some heavenly being, or maybe just checking the weather, and then he caught my eye. "I can't figure out why the field is so muddy. It doesn't make sense," he called out, waiting for a response, as if I would have an answer. I just shrugged.

"I'll be back. Going to get the diesel and tow it," he said.

The diesel truck would rip up the lawn, but there was nothing else to be done. I looked around. Dusk was tucking in around the farm; the mosquitoes were beginning to swarm, the crickets were serenading one another, the birds were finding their way to their nests. Within minutes Chris was back, securing a rope to the tractor.

By the time he had hitched it to the truck, it was pitch black out. Only headlights illuminated the dark field, and I could no longer see Chris's face. The truck engine roared to life and I waited on my lounge chair to see if this experiment would work. The next sound was the now familiar whir of tires spinning hopelessly in the mud, only this time it was not the mower. The truck was stuck, too. I did what any supportive wife and self-respecting pregnant city girl would do in this situation. I busted open a huge bag of popcorn and called Watson to give him a play-by-play.

Chris must have heard me talking, because he stopped what he was doing and looked up. "Who are you talking to?"

"Watson. He wants to know if you thought about the fact that the truck might get stuck since the tractor got stuck."

"Oh yeah?" He was not amused.

"I didn't say that," insisted Watson.

"Better it come from you than me."

"What's he doing now?"

"I think he's trying to push the truck. Should I ask?"

"Do you value your life?"

"We'll all laugh about this someday. We're making memories," I said.

"Bizarre farm equipment memories. You know this doesn't happen to people in Brooklyn, right? COME HOME."

"That's because people in Brooklyn don't have lawns."

"That is exactly my point. How's the baby?"

"Good. Doctor says he or she is the size of a small butternut squash and growing."

"Yeah, that's another thing that doesn't happen in Brooklyn. We don't measure babies in vegetables. We use something called numbers."

Pellets of hail began to fall; luckily, I was protected by our gigantic deck umbrella. I called down to Chris, "Can I get you anything? An umbrella, maybe?" We didn't own any umbrellas, other than the one on our deck, but I was trying to be helpful.

"No, Mike is coming to help. I just got off the phone with him."

Minutes later a large white pickup came tearing through the grass, headlights blazing. Mike, a local landscaper, climbed down from his truck to assess the situation. The two men stood in the field as the hail turned to pouring rain, hands on their hips, shaking their heads back and forth.

"What are they doing?" Watson wanted to know.

"They're staring at the tractor. Why do men do that staring thing?"

"You mean thinking?"

"Wait, Mike is getting a really big chain out of his truck. Do people just have those things lying around?"

"Maybe he's into bondage."

"It's really thick."

"Maybe he's into bondage with things other than people. You live in the country."

"You're disgusting."

"Moooo."

Instead of trying to dislodge the tractor, they focused on freeing the truck. Chris pushed as Mike hauled. At some point there was plywood involved, and also cursing. Fifteen tire-spinning, mud-flinging minutes later, the truck was free.

"Four-wheel drive, baby!" Mike hooted as the two made their way to the house doing some sort of male victory dance.

"What about the tractor?" I called out from the deck. The men turned to look at me and then back at each other, their moods palpably sinking. "I mean, I'm just asking because Watson wants to know."

"Bitch," Watson said from the other end of the receiver.

"Ran out of gasoline with all that revving. Going to come back for it tomorrow," Chris said, continuing toward the house, mud swathed across his face and dripping from his boots. I made my way back to bed and heard him rummaging through the refrigerator.

The next day Chris called me from work to tell me that the tractor was stuck because the ground was too wet. It must have been his keen powers of observation that had so drawn me to him. He said the ground wasn't supposed to be that wet but he had a sneaking suspicion about the reason. Also, he thought it might cost a lot of money to fix so he wanted to prepare me.

Not long after, I heard the sound of the diesel cutting to a halt in the driveway. Satchie Red's tail began wagging, but when Chris didn't come in the house, both the dog and I looked out the window to see that he was knocking on our tenants' doors. Pop had converted the cow barn into a four-family apartment complex in the eighties, and the tenants, who were all pretty much recluses, had been living there longer than we had. I had never been inside any of their apartments. Come to think of it, I had only seen each of them a handful of times.

Either Chris had secret plumbing knowledge he'd never told me about or, more likely, he had talked to someone about plumbing. Somehow he had figured out that the source of the mysterious backyard swamp was inside one of the barn apartments. Three of the tenants came up clean, but then he knocked on the door of the fourth. The tenant insisted that there was no leak in the apartment, but Chris sweet-talked his way in to have a look.

When he reappeared, he was pale and visibly shaken. He'd seen all sorts of makeshift home repairs before; hell, he'd even seen a car frame holding up his own basement ceiling. But nothing had prepared him for what he found in that tenant's bathroom. A long, slimy, rotten broom handle was jacked up into the cold-water tap of the bathtub faucet and duct-taped around partly exposed piping. The mechanism for the knob had been stripped, and the tenant was using the broom handle to turn the water on and off. When Chris removed the broom handle, water came pouring out. The tenant said it was nothing, he didn't want to be a bother, it was a little leak, had only been a problem for the last *five years*. But it was leaking not only into the tenant's bathtub; it was also leaking into the yard. And it wasn't little!

The next day a very expensive plumber dove headfirst into a deep hole in my backyard while his assistant held his legs straight up in the air. The strap of his blue overalls had come undone and was dangling down, or should I say up, the length of his body. Aside from the lawn mower fiasco, this was the most excitement I'd had in months. It was confirmed that all the water was pouring into the leach field and flooding about six acres of our land.

Lying in my lounger on the deck that evening, as the sky slowly darkened over the valley, I saw that sad and lonely tractor still sitting in the field. I listened hard; just above the clamor of the crickets, it was my father's voice. "You're in deep, kid."

21 | Dream Crusher

Chris was gone. He was sitting on the pink-and-blue-striped chair in the living room, his shoulders squared, but he was gone. His long fingers strummed the armrest. I had seen that look before.

Junior year of high school, my father had quit his job again. He'd had a disagreement with his boss and was back on the couch; only now it was pastel with a soft floral pattern, no plastic. My grandmother began buying us food, and likely paying the rent, and when I checked my savings account to see if I had enough money for a new leather motorcycle jacket, I saw it had been drained. My father had taken it. It was an act of desperation to pay the bills, but my teenage self could only see the betrayal, and I found no sympathy for him. When I approached him, he was sitting in the living room in his pink velvet rocking chair, my mother having long since thrown out his Archie Bunker chair. He didn't respond to my inquiry. Instead, he looked past me, like Chris was now, contemplating his next move. Then with soft eyes, he pleaded with me not to tell my mother, but I was so hurt that I didn't even consider it. They fought for days.

When I asked my mother for the details of that incident, she said, "Your father had gone from being flush with cash and showered with colored televisions and designer clothing as a buyer who brought in multimillion-dollar deals, to sneaking around in his children's rooms and cashing out their savings to pay the electric bill." That is a long way for a man to fall. I pressed her to go on, but she said, "It still pains me to talk about it, to try to sort it out, to think about how I could have done something different so my own husband didn't feel compelled to take from our children."

For months after, my father and I hardly spoke. I was no longer a little girl and now he embarrassed me in front of my friends. He wore the same clothes for days, and didn't care much for showering. When other kids asked where he worked, I lied, telling them he was still a dispatcher at Busy Bay Bee.

Now I studied Chris's face, his full lips pursed in contemplation. I knew how to get him back. I could swing my legs over the bed, get up, and walk away from this voluntary confinement. I could fix our finances and our marriage. I could rent and paint the apartments, work at the shop, start freelancing again. But to do so would be risking the life of our unborn child.

He stood up and went into the kitchen, and in his place, I saw a faint outline of my father, eyebrows askew, his flyaway comb-over falling into his milky eyes, the three-day stubble on his sunken jowls. "This is not Brownies. You don't get to quit on my grandchild. Kabeen, I'm warning you." He raised his eyebrows as if to challenge me.

"Why not? You quit everything. You quit almost every job you ever had."

"That was different. "

"Bullshit. What was different?"

"I want you to be better. "

"Well, you should have thought about that back then."

"I did. Every day. I quit a lot of things, Kabeen. But I never quit you." It was true. We went through contentious years, and he gave up jobs, money, dreams, but he never gave up on me.

It seemed that whatever decision I made would be the wrong one. Maybe I wasn't the capable woman I had professed to be.

I knew I had to protect my child, but at what cost to my marriage? I wanted to help Chris, but I couldn't find a way to do that without endangering the baby.

"I'm going for a drive," Chris called out. I'd hoped he would come sit next to me so we could work through this together. But he didn't come home until long after I had gone to sleep.

It was still July. I couldn't believe it was still July. The days had stopped. I would go to sleep on a Monday and wake up and it would still be Monday. Hours and hours that just didn't move, like a sloth in the blazing summer sun. The only way to shift this stagnation was to set mini goals and revel in small accomplishments because thinking of the long, slow march to the very last days of September was a grueling prospect. I thought only about getting through another day, about Josephine coming to clean, about my massage therapist, and maybe a visit from Jackie.

Chris was having a hard time seeing the finish line, too.

"What if you gave this all up and went back to jiu-jitsu?" I asked him when he came home from work in a better mood than the night before.

"I can't. Those days are over."

"I want you to be happy."

"I have to support us. It's all on me right now."

"It's like if I had to give up writing. I couldn't do it. Fighting was your life."

"I can't think about jiu-jitsu now."

On our first date Chris had mentioned he was a fighter, but I had assumed it was just a hobby. Then on the car ride home from our first Christmas together, I found out the real story when I asked him about his mother.

"Are you guys close? It's hard to tell."

"When I was younger. But after college we started disagreeing about some choices I made, so we grew apart."

I waited to hear more.

"As a kid, we'd do cool stuff together. She'd take me to high tea at the Waldorf, or find fresh strawberries in the middle of winter and make a big deal of whipping up cream. But then I got older. I began to really focus on jiu-jitsu, and she didn't like it."

One day he strolled into a local studio and discovered he had a unique talent for beating the crap out of people. That's when they began calling him the Sandman and his prowess got him an invitation to live and train in Brazil. He entered multiple competitions and did well, but he had to come back for medical treatment after a year, when he couldn't shake off an infection in his elbow.

"So you gave it up?" The more I got to know Chris, the more complex he seemed. When we were dating I remember thinking that I wanted to spend the rest of my life peeling away the layers, revealing what was beneath that quiet exterior.

"I came home and opened an academy in Philly. I couldn't make money. My mom was on my case. She wanted me to get what she considered a real job. So I did. My mother blames everything that ever went wrong in my life on jiu-jitsu."

"But it's your *passion*," I said. How do you just give up the thing you love the most?

"Yeah. I know." He watched the road ahead of him and didn't speak for a while.

How much power could someone have over her grown child that she could stop him from doing what he loved? I couldn't tell if it was about money, or maybe she was worried that he'd get hurt. Later I would understand that it was both.

Now, I propped myself up on my pillows and said, "I think it would be good for both of us if you started training again. You need an outlet for all the stress." Even though he had put it on the back burner, I thought if I could nudge him in that direction and let him know I supported it, he might consider the possibility.

He came over to the sofa, chewing a granola bar, and lowered his gaze to meet mine. "Yeah, wish I could."

"We'll make it work."

He turned away.

I blamed myself. He hadn't trained once since I began bed resting. I could see a parallel between Chris's jiu-jitsu dreams and my father's plan to be a private investigator. I'd lived with my father's regret all my life, and I didn't want to live with Chris's now.

"Take a day, go to New York City and train at your old studio."

"Here's the thing about training." He turned toward me. "You don't just start fighting after not fighting. You can't just walk into a studio and get your ass handed to you. You walk through that door and you need to be ready, ready to show them that nothing has changed, that you're still who you've always been."

"Words to live by," I whispered, nodding mostly to myself.

"I'm going to work on the renovations," he added before disappearing.

I lay there absorbing the power of what he had just said. *Nothing has changed; you're still who you've always been.* Just because I had to stay in bed didn't mean I was now worthless. It didn't change who I was. Deep down, I was still strong. I was just having a hard time tapping into that right now. But keeping our baby safe was as important as the business and the apartments and the bills, maybe even more so, because all that other stuff, that was *for* our baby.

"Have you thought about my mother's offer?" Chris said, reappearing from scraping wallpaper. He was talking about a baby shower. Just a few months ago, I had coveted so many baby items: the blue treasure box at Tiffany for baby's first lock of hair, the silver-plated teddy bear bank, the chic diaper bags.

"Who needs all that stuff anyway?"

"What'd you do with my wife?"

I didn't answer. Mostly because I wasn't sure. Try as I might to conjure the desire, I no longer felt the need for these trinkets. "Our baby, if we indeed *have* this baby, will be lucky if it has a onesie," I said, turning to face the wall.

I had been nudging aside whispers of showers and parties. My mother-in-law, Nadine, practically begged me to put together a registry. She enticed me with sweet impractical items, generously offering up the much-coveted and backordered Bugaboo stroller. I said no, I didn't want it, and somewhere inside me a little fashion diva curled up and died.

There would be no false optimism here. I couldn't wrap my mind around the absolute horror of having baby items in the house when we still weren't sure the outcome would be positive. The thought of dismantling a whole room of what should have been was too much to bear, but my anxiety forced me to play it out anyway. I imagined Chris doing it by himself, throwing boxes of baby clothing, diaper dispensers, and cute fuzzy blankets down the stairs into the Basement of Death and Despair, where it would remain until he could bring himself to dispose of it.

Admittedly, there was this little hopeful party girl inside me that would not have minded wearing a goofy shower hat made of ribbons; I just wasn't sure I could handle it.

Chris went back to scraping, so I called my mother to feel her out, expecting her to convince me to go for it.

"Don't do it," she said. The woman never ceased to surprise me. "Jews don't have baby showers."

For a split second I thought maybe I really did want a shower.

"No reason to tempt fate. Pooh pooh pooh," she said. I knew she was holding her index and middle fingers together and spitting on them three times to ward off evil.

My mother had solved my problem. Jewish girls don't have baby showers. I would explain to my mother-in-law that though I understood this was supposed to be a celebration honoring me and the baby, I would follow in the footsteps of my Jewish sisters and wait until after the baby was born before commencing festivities. Sometimes it's okay to play the Jew card. Not long after I hung up the phone with my mother, Chris stood in front of me covered in dust.

"I would like to meet the person who invented wallpaper. It's like tattooing your walls. You can never get rid of it."

"We could always tear down the house and build a new one."

I'd spent many nights in bed listening to Chris scraping. The unceasing rhythmic sound was like Poe's "Tell-Tale Heart." Sometimes, even after Chris was done for the evening and lying in bed beside me, I could still hear the scraping. Maybe it wasn't scraping at all. Maybe it was something under the floorboards. I made a mental note to discuss it with Watson.

Chris invited me to see his progress. I had to think about whether I had the energy. Because it would take a while to gather myself together, he told me to meet him in the master suite. I was excited at the prospect of seeing what had been accomplished.

I turned onto my left side, allowing the contents of my uterus to readjust. I wrapped both hands around the underside of my belly and gently heaved it up. Then I swung my legs over the bed and stood. I waited for my hips to find their place before beginning the slow shuffle forward. Just as I could see the finish line, the door to the suite, a monstrous wolf spider scurried out from under the bookshelf in the hallway.

I belted forth a primal scream. "Satchie Red, kill!" She sniffed the floor in the general area but, unimpressed, turned away. The dog eats deer poop, but it offended her sensibilities to consider a wolf spider. I backtracked to the kitchen and grabbed a can of Raid from under the counter.

"Hold your breath, little fetus," I said, and then dispensed three-quarters of the bottle into the environment, single-handedly destroying the ozone layer once and for all. Baby spiders that had been hanging on to their mother's back scurried across the floor. I stumbled backward, screaming and shooting the can in all directions until the entire room was filled with fog. When I was sure I destroyed the last of them, I stopped. "Oh no, I just killed the babies. We never kill the babies. Not even little spider babies." But there was no taking it back. Their carcasses lay curled up in front of me. I took a deep breath and the scent of the Raid made me woozy. I ran to Chris, ready to fall into his arms and confess that I had just screwed up the cycle of life and likely jinxed our family. I stopped short.

"What are you doing in your underwear?" I said, taking another deep inhalation, this time being met with wallpaper-remover fumes. Was there no fresh air in this house?

Chris was standing there in his tighty-whities, scraping away a small square patch of wall. Sweat was dripping down his back, the old radio blaring Eddie Money's "Two Tickets to Paradise," the small lamp on the floor barely illuminating the big room.

"It is hot as blazing hell in here," Chris said. "This stuff is like Bondo. It's real glue. Before regulations. I need a flame-thrower. We have layers of wallpaper from every decade." I came closer, bits of paper swirling around me. There were big red flowers, tiny blue flowers, gold stars. Gold stars? Who has wallpaper with gold stars? Why was there so much wallpaper?

"Maybe we can hire someone," I whispered, but he didn't acknowledge it. Chris was an island of self-sufficiency. No man would come into his castle and take away the privilege of rebuilding his homestead, the land generations of his kinfolk had toiled over. "Is there any way to make this easier?" At this rate we'd be here until our child was in an old folks' home. "Is there anything we can do?" I tried again. Scrape, scrape.

I turned away from Chris and surveyed the room. That's when I said it. "How is it possible that in all the time you've been here, you've only scraped about one square foot of wallpaper?"

The moment those words left my lips, I regretted them. Chris paused, then continued working. I watched a gold star spiral to the floor, and then skulked out of the room and back to bed. Not only couldn't I help, but every word I uttered made things worse. It was the story of my life.

When I was twelve, we received a call that my paternal grandfather had died. My parents threw their coats on and fled out the door. Mark and I spent the rest of that evening sitting on the hallway floor, waiting for them to come home. It's not lost on me that fifteen years later, my brother and I chose that very same spot to spill our grief when my father died, as if every other room in the house were too bright and well decorated.

My father hadn't shed a single tear for his father. Come to think of it, I never saw him cry about anything. The day of my grandfather's funeral, my father paced back and forth in the dining room, absently rubbing his hands together. I had never seen him so agitated.

Not knowing how to comfort him, I blurted out, "Where are we having Thanksgiving this year?"

He turned to me, his face red, and shouted, "I don't give a damn about Thanksgiving. My father just died." I was stunned, the force of his words physically pushing me backward, but he wasn't finished. "What the hell is wrong with you?" he roared. I was consumed by guilt, knowing I had made a mistake and wishing I had just kept quiet.

If I could change any single moment in my relationship with my father, that's the one I would choose. I'd run across the room and throw my arms around his stout body. I would cry into his chest and let him soothe me, and in that way, he would be allowed to acknowledge his own grief. I would tell him, "I'm sorry, Daddy. I'm so, so sorry."

Instead, I am left with the memory of him standing in the dining room, the same way I had stood in the funeral home when it was time to bury him, surrounded by people but desperately alone, the same way I felt now, here on bed rest mourning the loss of my autonomy and the beautiful relationship I once had with my husband. Perhaps I was being melodramatic. Bed rest was temporary and my baby was hanging on, but the ache in my heart was the same.

A few days after my grandfather's Shiva was over, my father got up from his usual spot on the living room floor and said, "Well, Kabeen, you lost your grandfather a lot younger than I lost mine." That was all he ever said to me about his father's death. It was the fewest number of words he could use to acknowledge my own grief, and it meant everything.

I fell asleep to the sound of the scraper, with tears streaming down my face, and when I awoke in the morning, Chris was already gone. He hadn't even come to bed. Midday, he stopped home from work and ran directly to the bathroom without saying hello. I could hear him retching. He reappeared with a glassy look in his eyes, and I knew he had hit the proverbial wall. He mumbled something about the mechanics giving him grief at the shop and inhaling too much wallpaper glue, and then he disappeared back into the bathroom. I called out to him from the sofa bed, "You okay in there?"

He opened the door, this time to get a glass of water, supporting himself on the kitchen counter. "It's time to call Scary Larry," he croaked and ran back to the bathroom.

22 | Sandman Rising

Week 29½

Scary Larry lived in a run-down shack with car parts and beer bottles strewn across his front yard. Word on the street (or backcountry road as the case may be) was that he had an unsavory reputation. Scary Larry had been arrested on more than one occasion for disturbing the peace, and he definitely wasn't someone you wanted to meet in a dark alley. I don't make a habit of letting people like Scary Larry into my house.

Yet, because a customer at the shop insisted he was both good and cheap, Scary Larry was now standing in front of me: tall and skinny, greasy black hair, smelling of alcohol. Chris led him into the master suite and I followed. This was worth getting out of bed for. As Chris spoke, Scary began pacing the room. He was mumbling something I didn't catch. His hands were shaking. He pulled a single cigarette out of his shirt pocket. "You can't light that," I said. He didn't answer. Instead, he left it dangling from his dry lips.

As Chris began showing Scary how little progress had been made in peeling the wallpaper, Scary Larry reached for something hidden in the back of his pants. He jerked around and the next thing I knew, he was holding up a huge hammer and walking toward Chris. I backed closer to the door. Chris had his back to Scary. I willed him to turn around. "Chris!" I said, but he was still talking. Scary was inches from Chris when he raised his hammer and slammed it into the wall right by Chris's head. Then he did it three more times. The wall crumbled.

Just like that. I picked my jaw up off the floor and watched as Chris let out an uneasy laugh.

"Wallpaper's gone. Got a broom?" Scary looked at us.

That was one way to solve the problem.

He spent the rest of that afternoon putting up Sheetrock but didn't spackle. He had also agreed to do the floors. They were worn and in desperate need of sanding and re-staining. But then Scary Larry disappeared. After three days I had a feeling he wasn't coming back. I guess that's what you get when you hire a guy who goes by the first name of Scary. I had tasted the sweet nectar of productivity and there was no going back. "Hang in there, little butternut squash. We'll find someone to fix this place up before you get here," I said, patting my round belly.

When Josephine arrived, I told her our predicament as she made her way across the room with a dry mop. She wasn't supposed to be here until next week but had just shown up and started cleaning, and I wasn't about to stop her. I think she knew how lonely I was. She suggested we hire her husband, Sam, to sand and stain the floors.

I needed to strike while the iron was hot—that is, before Chris changed his mind about enlisting help. A half hour later an elfish-looking man with a long scraggly beard came sauntering in. His fee was reasonable and he claimed to have experience with a floor sander. I was sold. I called Chris and asked him to rent a sander from the hardware store and then come home to work out the details. The sander whirring around the wood floors was the sweet sound of progress, and even though it was a small act, I was smugly proud of myself for facilitating it.

Feeling that my work here was done for the day, I clicked on the television, shifting around to find a comfortable position in the August heat. I found a marathon of cooking shows about desserts for kids' birthday parties and watched in horror for two straight hours as they added excessive amounts of sugar into the batter for cupcakes, ice-cream cones, and mini cakes. Halfway through the third show, I dialed Watson.

"When I have this baby, I will never let him eat sugary crap."

"Did you hear what you just said?"

"Oh, I know all parents say that sort of thing, but I mean it."

"No, what you said about your baby."

"Yeah, when I have this baby—"

"That was it. You said it again. I'm so proud of you."

"What?"

"You exhaust me. Pay attention. You said *when*. Not *if*. Congratulations."

"I guess I did."

"I have to go. And by the way, your kid is *so* going to eat sugar."

I smiled. As I was hanging up, I heard a screech followed by a loud crash.

I did not want to know.

I rolled myself into a seated position, grabbing the sheets for leverage, and made my way to the master suite with turtle-like stealth, cursing my naive self for not asking for references. I had a feeling that whatever was behind the door to the master suite was going to cause great animosity between me and Chris. Unwilling to commit to stepping inside, I peeked into the room. I gasped aloud and my hands flew over my mouth in horror. A large section of the floor was sanded all right. Practically down to the joists. There were huge gouges in the floorboards.

Dust swirled through the air. The sander was on its side. Sam the Elf was sitting in the corner smoking a cigarette and shaking his head. Why did all these people think it was okay to smoke in a pregnant woman's home?

"Isn't that interesting? I've never seen a floor like that. It must be a pattern underneath the old wood." He pointed his cigarette in the direction of the divots, his beady little black eyes darting back and forth from me to the sander. Josephine peered in, shrugged, and announced she was going to a doctor's appointment. She would be back later in the afternoon to finish up.

I was no expert, but this did not seem right, and that was no pattern. Not knowing how to respond, I closed the door and got back into bed. Holding the phone in my hand, I hesitated. It was going to ruin his day. I was tired of being the one who always ruined his day. I was a needy pregnant wife who couldn't drive to the store, couldn't find a decent contractor, couldn't even keep a baby inside her own belly without it being a huge production. I hated myself. But I had no choice. There was a guy sitting amid a dust shower in our half-renovated bedroom, we were paying him by the hour, and my only hope of salvation was that he might drop that damn cigarette he shouldn't have been smoking in the first place and burn down the whole house.

I dialed.

"You might need to come home," I said. I could hear the hustle of the shop and a few thick, heavy voices. Landscapers, I thought.

"Hold on." He put down the phone to finish up with a customer. When he picked up again, he said, "How can I help you?" forgetting it was me.

"You can take me out back and shoot me. Just throw me on the woodchuck pile."

"Too easy. What's going on?"

"The floor is having issues. If I try to explain it, my blood pressure will skyrocket and my head will explode. There will be blood on your lovely seventies wood paneling. Please come home and deal with it?"

I tried to remember what made me think it would be fun to live in an old run-down farmhouse. You read about this type of thing in the *New York Times* all the time: hipster couple gives up their much-sought-after-but-too-small-for-a-growing-family-industrial-loft-style apartment, quits their corporate jobs, falls hopelessly in love with a fixer-upper in the country, charmed by the shopkeepers who chat with you while taking twenty minutes to ring up three grocery items, and they decide they'll raise goats for cheese to sell on Sundays at the local farmers' market for forty-five dollars a pound. I wanted to be those hipsters. I wanted goats, damn it. Or llamas. I wanted the *New York Times* dream. But there's something the *New York Times* doesn't tell you. If they ever did a follow-up article, they would find that after maybe two years, those very same people are bankrupt and on the verge of divorce. They're fighting over their goats in court. The man has embraced the country life: dresses in plaid, big work boots, chops more wood than he'll ever need. But he can't get the cheese business up and running, and the woman is hightailing it back to the city for a buttery croissant at Zabar's. That old show *Green Acres* was more documentary than sitcom, and I was living it.

Chris was home minutes later. Sam the Elf had not, as I had hoped, burned the house down. I waddled behind Chris but was jolted by a sharp stabbing pain in my belly. I tried to breathe through it. This was not the usual pain. This was something else. I froze. *Please don't let this be labor. We are doing so well.* Chris didn't notice that I was no longer behind him, and I just stood there, waiting to see what would happen next. Maybe it was just gas. Maybe the Monsters were rebelling. Maybe it was God's way of saying, "Hey, things could always get worse." The pain dulled, and within a few moments it passed, though I stood there for an extra minute just to be sure. Okay then. Weird, but everything seemed to be back to my normal level of discomfort.

I found my stoic husband listening to Sam's story about the unique patterns under the wood. Chris showed no emotion. His lips were a thin line and his gaze direct. It was this very face that made him intimidating to others. No one in the world could read him the way I could. It was a face that said, "You just ruined the floors that my grandfather built with his bare hands. You'll never set foot in my house again."

"Just stop working for now," Chris said quietly. "I have to think about this." He turned, kissed me on the forehead, and said, "I gotta get back to work." I went back to my bed, rummaged around for my tiara, positioned it on my head, and consulted Google to learn a thing or two about sanding. I discovered that when you sand floors, you must keep the sander moving at all times. You cannot hold the sander in one place to answer your cell phone, light a cigarette, adjust your crotch, or admire the view. You must move evenly and steadily from one end of the floor to the other without pausing.

Chris made some calls, and soon he reappeared with another contractor. This one seemed to actually know how to use a sander.

"Thousand bucks, I can fix this mess. That's just for one room. The other one will cost you another five hundred. Plus materials."

I wish I were a fainter; if I were a fainter, I'd have been flat on the floor, but instead, I had to hold myself up against the doorjamb and watch Chris's shoulder's slump in defeat. Unfortunately, Josephine, who had recently come back to finish up her cleaning for the day, was none too happy to see another contractor taking over her husband's job. She dropped her bucket of water and it splattered on the floor. "You can't do this. This is Sam's job."

Josephine wasn't Martha Stewart, but she was good enough, and the unspoken rule of domesticity is that when you find a housekeeper you like, you agree to sign over the mortgage to your house if she so desires. But there was no placating her, and in one fell swoop I lost not only a second contractor but a perfectly entertaining housekeeper. She gathered her mop and bucket and out of a final act of compassion said, "I'll clean this floor, but then I'm leaving. You have some nerve. You rich people are always taking advantage."

I was shocked that this was how she saw us. We were drowning in debt, we couldn't catch up on our bills, but she perceived us as well-off because we owned a business and a house. Chris had taken risks that we hoped one day would pay off. He had a determination to succeed that I had never seen. Growing up, we never owned a home, we didn't go on vacations, and I went to college on financial aid and loans. That's where I came from, that's who I was. But suddenly I had more assets than I ever dreamed of, and to Josephine, we were wealthy.

Chris was back in the pink-and-blue-striped chair tapping his fingers. I was trying to make eye contact, but he didn't notice. I knew he was wondering where the fifteen hundred dollars was supposed to come from. If I tried to comfort him, it would come out all wrong and we would fight, so I stayed quiet while he tapped.

He picked up the phone to call his client Tom; Chris had been Tom's real estate agent before taking over the shop. They still had one big deal pending, and now it was time to push for a closing. Tom was Chris's golden goose. They used to do jiu-jitsu together, and when Tom first walked into the real estate office looking for an agent to help him buy land in the booming real estate market a year before, it was pure luck that Chris was at his desk and not out showing houses to tourists who had nothing better to do. There was no question the two would work together. For a while Chris closed one fat juicy deal after another, but just as quickly as the Hudson Valley had become *the* place to be, the economy began to tank. It was only the beginning, but anyone who was paying attention could see that the bubble was about to burst.

Chris got up to wash dishes in the kitchen while he spoke to Tom, but I could still hear Chris's side of the conversation.

He tended not to share too much information with people, so I was surprised to hear him telling Tom that I was on bed rest. Of course, my general greeting to anyone who called was: "Nice to hear from you, I'm on bed rest. Let me tell you about my incompetent cervix and my Monster Fibroids." But that wasn't Chris's modus operandi.

Then Chris began explaining to Tom *why* I was on bed rest. Here were two men who tore each other limb from limb for sport, and Chris was saying, "I guess we have fibroids." My breath caught. He said *we*. My husband, the Sandman, the guy who kicks people in the face for fun, said, "*We* have fibroids." They were ours. He was sharing my fibroids. I laughed, and I almost cried, too. He had, in his own way, taken on my burden as his own. I sang it in my head over and over. *We have fibroids. WE have fibroids.*

While I listened to him describe the pressure of the Monsters on my cervix, I reveled in the love I had almost forgotten was there. I knew I'd have to do something to show him I still loved him, too.

23 | Battle on Cervix Hill

Week 30

The seductress of Ulster County had risen. I ordered a book, and it had nothing to do with pregnancy. This little piece of mail-ordered merchandise was going to change the arid desert of our love to a lush landscape of amorous escapades. The book had secret sealed pockets, and inside each little pocket was a spicy challenge. The titles on the pockets were cryptic and enticing: "Winner Takes All," "South of the Border," "The Velvet Hammer." I showed the book to Chris.

"The deal is, you open your secret pocket and I open mine, and we do what the instructions say, no matter what."

"What if it says to jump in front of a semi?"

"Love knows no bounds." I smiled. "Now, go away and open yours, do what it says, and fall madly, desperately in love with me all over again."

"I'm desperate, all right," he said, grabbing his secret pocket.

As soon as he left the room, I peeled open the one that said "For Her Eyes Only" and read the title: "The Do-Me Decimal System." The words "What do men *really* want?" were printed directly underneath. This was going to be easy. Men want peace and quiet. A secretary. A car that has the ability to go in reverse. More sleep.

Inside the pocket, along with directions, was a Love Coupon to be saved for a later date. Once I gave this coupon to Chris, he was supposed to be under my spell for fifteen minutes and do whatever I say. I took that to mean that for fifteen minutes

I could have him scrub the kitchen floor and he couldn't complain. The Do-Me Decimal System instructed me to take my partner to the library to pick out articles about the day he was born. That was supposed to make him feel special, and then he would ravage me right there among the stacks. Except our library was in an old stone house with squeaky floorboards that didn't quite lend itself to passionate lovemaking. Plus, I couldn't go there because I was bedbound. But I *could* look up information online. The book promised this would make my partner feel loved and wanted.

When next I saw Chris, I set the seduction in motion. "Hey, did you know that your birthday is on the 206th day of the year?"

"Yeah?"

"Does that make you feel special?"

"No."

"Did you know that your birthday is the same day in history that the United States tested the first underwater atomic bomb?"

"Why are you telling me this?"

"And also, it's the world's first test-tube baby's birthday."

"What?"

"I'm being romantic."

"Oh. I must have missed that."

"It's what the book said to do."

"The book told you the world's first test-tube baby was born on my birthday?"

"Okay, what've you got?"

"You'll have to wait and see."

Chris walked away, and I was left wondering why my attempt to connect had fallen so flat. I had lost my edge. I had forgotten how to flirt. I was hoping to break through the barrier that had built up between us, maybe make him laugh, but nothing seemed funny anymore.

Produce Pete was on television talking about eggplant, and we were in the midst of a heat wave. As the temperature continued to rise, the house began settling in unsettling ways, creaking and moaning, not unlike myself. I was becoming the house. The house was me. It all felt very existential.

Even the usually cool country nights were sweltering. The slow, restless days dragged on and this house and I were on the verge of exploding. I could find no retreat. I waited to see what romantic idea Chris was going to come up with, but so far there was no trace of an advance. I was sure he had forgotten. Nothing of importance seemed to happen as I languished in bed, the world churning on without me, sadness my only bedfellow.

My eyes shot open. In my sleepy fog, I could almost make out the red-orange glow of the sunrise peeking through the window. Something was amiss. A sharp stabbing pain in my lower right abdomen forced me to take a harsh breath in. I'd dismissed it the first time a few days back, but now it was much more severe. I was so close to the finish line now. Only ten more weeks to go. I was afraid to breathe out. I pushed my sweaty, matted hair off my face. With another sharp pain, I braced for the worst and then placed my hand under the sheets to feel for blood. My hand came back dry. I turned to Chris, but he wasn't there. Holding back tears, I called out that we needed to go to the doctor now. He didn't hear me. He was on the other side of the house working on the renovations. I shouted his name in panic, but to no avail. Finally he appeared, ready to leave for work. I had already called the doctor, my face hot with fear.

Chris helped me to the car. He didn't say anything that would lead me to think he was concerned, but when he held my arm as I navigated the stone steps, he grabbed it so tight he cut off my circulation, and I knew he was as worried as I was.

I squirmed and wiggled, trying to contort my body into a comfortable position. Was this the culmination of all these months?

The baby leaving my body too soon? I hadn't been good enough after all. Tears welled not only for the pain but for my failure. I prayed to God and I struck a bargain with my father. "You will not let me lose this baby. I will not lose this child the way I lost you. If you do one last thing for me, keep this baby inside my body, alive. In return, I will pray for your eternal soul every day, lifting you up higher in the Lord's eyes." Suddenly I was a religious zealot, but I meant to keep my promise. Jews believe that each time you pray for a person's soul, it rises higher in heaven. I swore if this baby lived, I'd pray so hard that my father's soul would be catapulted right up to Yahweh's throne.

When we saw Dr. Enchanté this time, he was all business. He did not kiss my hand or entertain me with witty banter. After an ultrasound and an examination, he said, "The baby is fine. You're not miscarrying. Your fibroids are shrinking. There's a war going on in there."

I don't remember the technical terms Dr. Enchanté used, but he described a battle of wills between the Monsters and the baby for my blood supply, and even though the Monsters were putting up a hell of a fight, they were losing. The pain I was feeling was from the Monsters retreating. Instead of the tragedy I had anticipated, this was a small victory. It meant my little warrior was getting stronger. Dr. Enchanté told me that he would prescribe painkillers, but there was something about them being bad for the baby's kidneys, or liver, I couldn't remember which.

When I arrived home, my mother called from Port Authority for an update and to tell me she was on her way over. Chris had called her while I was getting dressed at the doctor's office. I got back into bed, relieved. Exhausted from both the morning's events and the excruciating pain, I fell into a fitful sleep.

Hours later I awoke to my mother standing over me with a ladle in her hand. "Aileen, take the pills."

"I'm not taking the pills."

"You can't just be in pain. Take the pills."

"I'm not going to damage my baby."

She hurried away in a huff, and soon I could hear her struggling to get the big stockpot out of the lazy Susan.

"I brought a chicken with me. I'll throw something together," she hollered.

I rolled over to stare out the bedroom window. If I took these pills, they would at best provide me with temporary relief, but there was a chance, however small, that my child would be born with two heads, or at the very least, half a liver. I had already given up most dairy (listeria), carbs (diabetes), and anything that tasted good (because, well, I was sure it would turn my child into a cyborg). Now painkillers had been scratched off the list, too.

"Talk to your brother," my mother said, throwing the phone onto the bed.

"I'm not taking the pills," I said, putting the receiver up to my ear.

"Take the pills," my brother said.

"Don't bully me." I scrunched up my face as another wave of pain washed over me.

"Nobody is bullying you."

"Dad would understand."

"Bad argument. He died because he was stubborn and didn't listen to his doctors."

"Why do you care if I take the pills?" I breathed out away from the phone.

"Because you're being selfish."

"My pain is selfish?"

"You're torturing your mother."

"So, you don't really care?"

"Only marginally. But it's time to take care of yourself now."

"I know you see it that way, but I've been fighting this war for months. This is just another skirmish. Why would I do something to screw up my chances now? Either way, it's going to suck. I can deal with the pain now, or I can spend a lifetime maybe regretting my decision."

After that, I thought of each stabbing rush as a win for my baby. I turned on chanting music and focused on breathing deeply, and it seemed to ease the pain.

"I brought you lunch. Eat." My mother put a plate of carrots and hummus on my tray. We had been butting heads since I was in high school. But now that I was about to become a mother, I was beginning to see that no matter the circumstances, no matter how stubborn or angry I became, this woman would always be there, always love me, and, as a bonus, I would never go hungry.

"Thank you."

"You're welcome." She stood there staring at me, waiting for me to take a bite.

Perhaps because I had come from a long line of Jewish women, I began thinking that the more I suffered, the more I would have a shot at keeping this baby alive. The waiting was almost over. I could deal with the pain.

I couldn't take the heat, though. I was on fire. That night I tossed and turned. There was something hard underneath my pillow. Half asleep, instead of looking for the culprit, I tried to roll my head away from it. Each time I'd drift off, I'd bump into it again. With eyes open and staring at the ceiling, I considered whether I wanted to pursue this knobby and unforgiving object, thinking that there was a very real possibility it was a petrified mouse. I rolled and threw my pillow to the ground, half expecting to find a carcass, but I couldn't see in the dark and I was afraid to put my hand there.

Squinting I could just see the outline of something grayish. I put one finger out and touched it. It was cold. It had to be a dead mouse. This is what happens when you live in the country; you find vermin under your pillow. I looked again but couldn't make out a face or limbs. Braver now, and with my curiosity piqued, I tapped it with the back of my hand.

It was a rock.

I picked it up and rolled it around between my palms, wondering if this had something to do with my mother's *bubbe-meises*, or old wives' tales. I turned it over, looking for a Hebrew inscription. The woman was always putting ribbons, index-card prayers, and Jewish stars under my mattress to ward off the evil eye. There were black words on the rock, but I couldn't make them out, so I put it on the nightstand, snuggled into my sheets, and threw my leg over Chris's body before falling back to sleep.

The next morning, in the light of day, I picked up the rock again, turning it over, and there, written with a Sharpie pen, were the words: "I love you, baby. You rock. Chris." I smiled. This was his thing.

24 | Helter Skelter Swelter

Week 30½

I reclined in bed while my mother stood with her back to me folding washcloths, the morning news blaring in the background.

"Mom, did you love Dad?"

"Sometimes more than others," she said without turning.

"Why did you stay with him?"

"You don't leave someone when they're down. And he was always down." She thought about it a moment longer. "He was a good man, mostly."

"What made you marry him?"

She turned to me then. "He made me feel safe." We remained silent for a long while as I rubbed my belly.

"What did Dad say when you told him you were pregnant the first time?"

"He said, 'Oh shit.' Then he went for a walk, came back, and was fine."

"That wasn't very supportive."

"He was very happy, but he was scared, too. That's how he dealt with it."

"Do you think he would have liked Chris?"

"I think they would have gotten along. As much as your father got along with anyone."

"What kind of thing is that to say?"

"Your father's whole goal in life was to be left alone."

"But you stayed."

"Where was I going to go?" She gathered the pile of wash-cloths, putting them in the laundry basket. "I really did love him, you know."

Then she headed to the linen closet, leaving me with my thoughts.

Jackie was at the door. I hadn't known she was coming, but here she was introducing herself to my mother, who was thrilled to meet one of my friends. They were chatting about foot cramps and potassium, and my mother was asking Jackie for the number of her orthopedic doctor. I looked down at my belly, knowing one day I, too, would embarrass my child, talk too much, and ask strangers inappropriate questions. I'd better get that meatball recipe so they'd keep me around.

"You probably don't want me here. I'll go into the other room," my mother said, turning to leave.

"Ma, you can stay."

"No, no, you visit with your friend. I'm happy to sit by myself." She turned and left.

"How's the pain?" Jackie said.

"Not so good, but better."

"Life is full of pain, sweetheart. I'm going to help you. One word. Visualization. Got that?"

"I may need another word or two."

"Relaxation techniques. It works. Half your pain is stress. There's nothing like a mental vacation to escape your uterus for a while." I raised an eyebrow and Jackie scooted herself up to the edge of the pink-and-blue-striped chair. Sitting up tall, she clasped her hands in her lap. "Take a deep breath. Find a place you want to go or a place you've been, and go there. Really go there. Get out of this stuffy house."

"I wish."

"Are you talking to your baby?"

"No."

"Oh, honey, you have to talk to your baby. Tell him what's going on. You never have to be alone. You have another person there right inside you. Soon they want nothing to do with you, trust me. My daughter isn't answering my calls. Right now, that baby is a captive audience." She pointed at my belly. "Don't you think the baby is wondering what's going on?"

I assumed my child thought the Monsters were its brothers and sisters—talk about sibling rivalry. I have a pretty intense relationship with my brother, but he never tried to steal my blood; he just tried to spill it as often as possible.

"I can't stay long. Doctor's appointment. Look at the size of my leg, all swollen." Jackie pulled up her black pant leg and showed me a heinous bruise the size of a small melon.

"What the hell, Jackie?"

"Phlebitis. Going now." She rummaged through her bag and pulled out a pack of cigarettes. Then she pointed at me, a cigarette now dangling between her two fingers. "Visualize. Do it. Report back. Feel better."

"Stop smoking," I yelled as she headed toward the door.

I moved to my lounge chair on the deck, taking with me three couch cushions to prop up and place between my legs. My yoga instructor had told me a story about a yogi who had been ill and bedridden, and so, to keep himself fit, he went through a series of yoga poses in his head. I took a few cleansing breaths, closed my eyes, and began my Sun Salutation, stretching up to the sky and swooping back down again to reach the floor, one foot back, and then the other. Plank, Chaturanga, and Upward Dog. I moved on to Warrior One and then Warrior Two. It was in this pose I felt most powerful, and so I stayed here. And then onto Triangle, and finally Pigeon.

It was working; I was deep inside myself. I hadn't moved this much in months. I was lighter. A truck pulled up to the house and cut its engine, breaking my concentration. Out stepped Dave, the Charlie Chaplin UPS guy. With a smile permanently glued to his face, and always bearing gifts, he was officially one of my favorite people. He came through the deck gate, his dark tight curls slicked back and neat, his collar open an extra button.

"Got a package for you." Satchie Red ran over to him, putting her two front paws up, muddying his beige uniform. "Can't fool this dog," he said as he reached into his pocket and pulled out a biscuit. Satchie Red looked at it, deciding if she would give him the satisfaction of accepting his offering.

"Hot today," I said.

He nodded.

"I mean the weather," I clarified. Oh my God, I had no idea how to talk to people anymore, especially men.

"Yeah. No air conditioner in the truck. Makes for a long day. At least I can look forward to it at home. Your dog doesn't like cookies?"

"She doesn't trust you, or anybody else for that matter."

"Well, I'll leave it here for her." He placed it on the ground and stepped away. Satchie Red ignored him. Charlie Chaplin and I had built up a sweet rapport, and over time I had learned tidbits about his route, his family, and his life. "Don't tell anyone," he said, leaning in, "but I might be up for a promotion. It would mean I wouldn't be on this route."

"I've got nine and a half weeks to go. You can't abandon me now. I'm in no condition to start over with someone new. Try to wait it out."

"Don't worry, I won't leave you high and dry. Tons of red tape. Hang in there. I'll see you in a few days."

Satchie Red followed him to the deck gate with her purple tongue lolling to one side. I watched her panting, the quick, deep intake of oxygen, the drool, her drooping jowls, and I suddenly had the most brilliant thought. It was something Charlie Chaplin had said. What was it? Oh, yes! Air-conditioning! We needed an air conditioner!

I dialed.

"Lawn and Power . . ."

"Do we own an air conditioner?" There was no time for hellos.

"What?" I didn't answer him. I could wait him out forever. I had no place to go. Finally, he broke. "We don't have an air conditioner. No one who ever lived in that house needed an air conditioner."

"The people who lived in this house didn't need support beams in their basement either. I'm ordering an air conditioner."

"You'll never find one that fits our windows."

"Is this a challenge?"

"We have jalousies, what the locals call trailer windows. They don't make an air conditioner that will fit those. Anyway, gotta go. Line of customers." I heard the phone click before I had a chance to say "I love you." I pictured Chris juggling three customers and the phone all at once . . . in an air-conditioned shop.

"Oh, it's on, baby!" I said to no one.

Chris's days were speeding up as mine slowed down. Everyone around me was constantly in motion. My mother couldn't sit still, and even Jackie only had time for short visits. What was so pressing? Where was everybody going? Had everyone always been this busy? Was I the only one who lay in the quiet stillness of the long afternoon listening to the birds, observing the same two hawks swooping over the field looking for a meal every single day? No one had time to notice the birds anymore. Satchie Red sniffed the biscuit Charlie Chaplin had left on the deck. She took one tentative lick and turned away, leaving it for the ants.

While my mother locked herself in the guest room with a fan and a pile of paperwork she had brought from home to sort through, I spent the rest of the afternoon becoming an HVAC expert. I already knew how to sand floors, could throw around some pretty impressive power-equipment jargon, and had figured out how to rent an apartment from bed. Now I was learning yet another skill that no one back in Brooklyn would ever believe. By the time I concluded my exhaustive search for cooling systems, I could have installed tubing for central air. Since that would never fly in this old house, I found one air conditioner with terrible reviews that would fit the small crank window in the formal living room.

If anyone had ever told me that true salvation comes in the form of a big brown UPS truck, I would have thought it was a lie. But a few days later, as I was sunning on the deck, there was Charlie Chaplin, shirtsleeves rolled up high past his biceps, sweat stains under his armpits. Even the fine, curled chest hairs peeking out of his uniform glistened. He walked up the deck steps, and the first thing I spied in the glaring sun was a faded rose tattoo on his forearm with the name "Linda" on it.

"Who's the lucky lady?"

"Sister . . . she died."

"Oh. Sorry."

"Long time ago." He shrugged. "Listen, there's no way this box is coming off the truck. Too heavy."

"It's an air conditioner."

"That explains it. I got a slipped disk." He placed his hand on his lower back.

I was so close to having cool air, I was salivating.

"Maybe you can help me pull it off the truck."

I cocked my head, biting my lower lip. I thought Charlie Chaplin and I understood each other. We had this great thing where he spoke and then I spoke, he gave me a present, and then he left. It was the perfect relationship. But now I felt like it had all been a lie. I wasn't even supposed to lift my lunch, let alone an air conditioner. How could he not know this?

"It's going to take about twenty minutes for me to even contemplate getting up from this lounger."

"Right. Maybe I can use that wheelbarrow over there?" I studied his features. He was older than I had thought. The lines on his face told a story. I didn't know if it was a story of sadness, resignation, or just hard living.

"How about this: leave it anywhere you like. My husband has superhuman strength. I've seen him lift a refrigerator by himself. He'll get it inside."

As he turned to go, I called to him. "Hey, any news about your promotion?"

"Nah, nothing yet. Don't worry, I won't leave you."

I smiled. "You deserve it, Dave. I hope it happens for you."

He nodded. "Thanks."

"Dave, do you like your job?"

"Yeah. You know, it's a job. I have a son."

"Preschool, right?"

"Yeah." He stood there, thinking. "I like to draw, make art. But you know, that don't pay the bills."

"What do you draw?"

"You see this tattoo? I designed it myself. Maybe I'll show you my work sometime."

"I'm going to miss you." And then I wondered if I shouldn't have said it. That is not what you are supposed to say to the UPS guy. But Dave had become much more than just a random stranger who brought me little pieces of happiness once in a while.

A few hours later, a screech followed by a bang stopped my mother in the middle of her lecture about the precision required to blacken a whole onion in a pan so that it flavors, but does not char, the chicken cutlets. "Fuck," I whispered. I threw my head back on the pillow and covered my eyes with my hand. Satchie Red strained her ears and ran to the window.

I cringed at the sound of the slamming screen door.

"There's a big box in the middle of the driveway," Chris said.

"I heard."

"Scratched up your car pretty good. Just the bumper though. We'll touch it up at the shop."

"Oh. Okay. Just the bumper? What about the box?"

"Just the bumper. The box is fine. Mostly grazed the wheelbarrow." He disappeared. Moments later I heard him struggling to fit the box through our narrow hallway, followed by a gentle thud.

"House isn't wired for this type of AC. Going to have to make a couple of calls." He placed it in front of the bed, where it would stay until we found someone to rewire the house.

Progress.

The next afternoon Chris came home with a buxom brunette and headed to the bedroom without stopping to say hello. There was nothing I could do. I wasn't even interested in watching. About ten minutes later, I heard the woman say, "I can't reach. Can you try to push it through the hole? I'll let you know when you're in." My eyes widened. I wished they would be quiet about it. But then I heard footsteps approaching. Maybe they were done.

Chris came in with the woman trailing behind. As she adjusted her work belt, I noticed her sculpted arms.

"This is Theo. She's working on the electric." Theo came over, extending her hand. Her skin was rough and her nails were raw around the cuticles. I tried not to be skeptical about the idea of a woman electrician. I wasn't worried about her electrical prowess; it was more the other kind of prowess I had concerns about. It is pure fact that men love women with power tools.

"Your wiring's shot. You plug that air conditioner into an outlet, probably blow up half the house."

Tempting.

The two of them worked together for the remainder of the afternoon, her pushing, him pulling, sparks flying, and finally we were ready for the great unveiling. Together they opened the box and pulled out the air conditioner. It was beautiful. I could almost feel the relief. Until Chris turned it around to face me. It was crushed on one side.

I put the back of my hand to my forehead. Defeated. Again. Perhaps I should have invested in a fainting couch instead.

25 | The Man behind the Curtain

Week 31

"You ready?" Chris called from the doorway. We were headed to Dr. Specialist for our routine sonogram. Maybe this time we'd get a more definitive answer about the sex of the baby.

"Pot roast for you when you get back," said my mother, pointing at Chris. "Aileen, you don't eat anything. Maybe a plate of celery." She kissed me goodbye, shooing us out the door.

I stepped out of the house and began the slow journey to the car, stopping every few steps to do a strange little dance. I wiggled my hips left to right and then thrust out my pelvis in jerky movements until bones, joints, and ligaments clicked into place. It felt like I was channeling Elvis.

Chris took a seat next to me in the waiting room, flipping through a *National Geographic* magazine. It bothered me that he was so relaxed, that he had no outward anxiety about our appointments. We could have used this time to talk, catch up, joke around, reassure each other, but instead, he had become more like a chauffeur than a husband, as much a stranger as everybody else in the room.

The techs knew me by now. I was the irrational one, the high-maintenance one who disagreed with her husband loudly in public places. The one who liked to argue over the existence of penises.

Stripped from the waist down. Paper robe. Cold gel. Husband seated behind me. We had the routine down.

"Okay. We're going to find out for sure. You ready?"

I strained my head back to look at Chris who nodded once. "We're ready," I said. Chris placed a firm hand on my shoulder while the tech glided the Doppler over my belly.

"Well, lookie there," she said, pointing to the screen. "That, my dear, is a penis."

I clapped my hands together. "Yes! I knew it!" I felt equal parts joy and vindication. I deserved a written apology from these nonbelievers . . . in glitter.

Chris squeezed my shoulder. He hadn't said it out loud, but I knew he wanted a boy.

Dr. Specialist came floating in, offering me a perfunctory hello before raising his glasses to his forehead to look at the scans. "Seems like we sorted out the baby's sex?"

"I knew we were having a boy," I said.

"How's the pressure on your cervix?"

Would no one give me the satisfaction of admitting they were wrong? "Slightly less unbearable, but there's still pressure," I replied.

"Well," he said, sitting down in a chair and rolling himself over to the screen. "Your fibroids have shrunk. Your pain should continue to lessen. It seems that everything is headed in a positive direction."

"I still hold the record for world's largest fibroid though, right?" He flipped through my chart. "I hear it's a coveted title," I tried again. Nothing.

"You don't need to be on bed rest anymore. You have to take it easy, but I don't see why you can't get up now."

"What?" Chris's disembodied voice came from behind my head. I parted my lips, but no words came out.

I made a few unintelligible sounds, and then blurted out, "Just like that?" Was this guy a magician? Did the barometric pressure shift? What had changed? I had a thousand questions.

"The truth is, I don't think you ever needed to be on bed rest."

"What?" Chris said again.

I brought my hand up to my cheek and slapped my own face. "I'm not understanding," I said.

"The fibroid was pressing on your cervix, but now it's shrunk so it's just pressing the side. It's actually keeping your cervix shut. You'll definitely need a C-section. You know that, right?"

"Um, I did not know that. I mean, I suppose with a Monster blocking the escape hatch, there's no other choice." Until now, I didn't even know for certain if there would be a baby. I had been trying so hard to keep it inside me; how could I possibly focus on its exit strategy?

"Well, there you have it. Anything else?"

Yes, there was something else. There were a billion some-things, but I couldn't articulate any of them in a way that would sound rational. What did he mean, he thought I never needed to be on bed rest? Why was he so flippant about it? I wasn't a statistic. You don't stop another human being's life for months and then say you didn't have to go through that, but no biggie, right?

As I got dressed, I tried to process the next steps. Could I just stop bed resting and pick my life back up like nothing had happened? This was what I had hoped for, what I had prayed for every day. And now that it was possible, all I wanted was to get back in bed and hide. I had the bed-rest version of Stockholm syndrome.

"Good news, right?" Chris said as he held the car door open for me.

"I'm not sure."

At home, I sat on the edge of the couch and held my belly. A voice inside me told me to ignore Dr. Specialist and lie back down, but I wasn't sure if that was instinct talking or fear. And I wasn't sure if it was my voice I was hearing, or my father's.

Two years before he died, my mother made him go to the hospital for chest pain. She called a cab, and they checked him in for a few nights. He was pissed. He hollered at everyone and refused to cooperate. My brother implored him to listen and to do what he was told, but he only responded, "I want to speak to my daughter. These doctors don't know what they're talking about." My brother called me at work and put my father on the phone. "Break me out of here, Kabeen." I told him I'd be over after work and we'd hatch a plan.

That night I stood at the edge of his hospital bed.

"You believe this shit?" he said.

"I can get you out of here. What's in it for me?"

"You'd bargain with your father? I'll take you out to Nino's." It was one of our favorite Italian restaurants, and we had recently started a little ritual of going out to dinner together once a month, just the two of us. Then, to sweeten the deal, he pulled out a small wad of cash and said, "Take what you want."

"Deal. But first you need some tests." I pocketed forty bucks and handed him back his cash. We both knew that he wasn't going anywhere, but I understood that he needed someone who would pretend with him. It was the only way he could accept sympathy. "I know you're fine, but these doctors can't release you until they're sure. So the quicker you sign the papers and take the tests, the quicker you're out of here."

When I was done talking, my mother came over with a wash-basin, pulled back the edge of the blanket, and washed my father's feet while he grumbled about how I was the only one who understood him. I will never forget the image of my mother standing there washing the man's feet while he yelled at her. When I asked her about it later, she said, "He was scared. He needed someone to yell at. After thirty years of marriage, you know when it's personal and when it's not."

My father never trusted doctors. He'd tell me not to listen to what they said and do what I thought was best. Then again, look where that got him.

My mother handed me a plate of sliced vegetables. "I can't talk about it, Ma," I cut her off before the interrogation began.

"Okay, fine. Chris told me, but I don't believe one word these *mamzer* doctors say. This one tells you one thing, the other says another thing. Call your OB. He'll tell you."

"You just said you don't believe anyone."

"Well, at some point you have to believe someone, right?" She waved her hand and left the room.

What would it mean to be liberated from bed rest? We were nearing the middle of August, and I had less than two months left to go. How would I fill that time? What about my hip dysplasia, the gestational diabetes? They weren't going to disappear. I didn't enjoy bed rest, but I was even more afraid of what would happen if I got up. I was like those prisoners who commit petty crimes just to get rearrested; I was safer on the inside. So taking my mother's Yiddishkeit logic into consideration, I called Dr. Enchanté and explained the new turn of events.

"You're so close. Why risk it? If you stop bed resting now and, say, deliver prematurely, you will have a much more diffi-cult road ahead. Now, that's not to say it won't happen anyway, but your course has been steady. It's almost, almost, but not quite, in the bag."

"Okay. So stay on bed rest?"

"Yes, I wholeheartedly disagree with the specialist."

"Well, there goes the gospel," I said mostly to myself.

"I'll give you this. You can have about an hour a day upright. Don't overdo it, but as long as you're not straining yourself, you can spend a small amount of time out of bed."

"Can I walk the dog in the yard?"

"Yes."

Mental high-five! "What about exercise?" I had become so weak and so soft that it was hard for me to imagine even lifting a baby. I needed to build some muscle.

He told me he would approve basic exercises like arm curls and leg lifts in moderation to keep the blood flowing and my muscles toned.

As soon as I got off the phone, I began doing reclined leg lifts. I had a new purpose. I was going to find my muscles. I started counting aloud, "One . . . two . . . one . . . two . . ."

"What are you doing?" My mother's panic-stricken voice echoed across the house.

"One, two, one, two, one, two." I sped up.

"Stop, you shouldn't be doing this."

"Ma, the doctor said it was okay. One-two-one-two-one-two." Even faster now.

"I don't agree with this."

"I'll get you a doctor's note. Will that be enough for you?"

"So you can't work out for a while. You think that's sacrifice? You should only know what I sacrificed for you."

"It's just a couple of leg lifts. I'm sorry that you had to sacrifice for me. I can't take it back. Okay?"

"I can't take it back either. Okay?"

"Okay."

"I'm glad we're all okay." She stormed out of the room, and I could hear my father's voice in my head, "Don't fight with your mother." He had said it a million times before, and he was right. Besides, I could see her point. You don't fold your son-in-law's underwear and not expect to at least get a healthy grandchild out of the deal. My mother was here to help, but we were in danger of falling back into old patterns. At least now I understood that this latest disagreement would blow over within approximately three minutes.

I stopped exercising and switched to visualization to lessen the strain on my mother's heart. This visualization exercise involved imagining blue beads slowly filling my body from head to toe, stretching muscles, tendons, skin, pelvis, torso, and chest. Toward the end of the exercise, the beads were supposed to spill out of my body and I would feel like putty. I pictured myself filled with beads. I was relaxing. It was great. But then the beads started multiplying. I couldn't keep up. I needed them out of my body. They were wrapping themselves around my throat. They were bearing down on my abdomen. And then, *bam!* I opened my eyes. The baby had kicked me right in the rib.

My mother was standing in front of me with her suitcase. She said she was all *schvitzed* out. It was too hot, too *meshuganeh,* she was getting the next bus home. "You'll be fine," she said. She leaned down and hugged me around my neck, which felt not unlike a choke hold, and then kissed me hard on the cheek, leaving a red smudge on my face. "I'll call you later. Maybe I'll come up again in the next week or two."

She pulled a chair up to the door, parked herself there, and waited for Chris to get home from work to drive her to the bus stop. She left us with a huge pot of brisket, enough chicken to last until my son's bar mitzvah, and a pile of Chris's neatly folded underwear.

26 | A Low Guttural Howl

Week 31½

Chris's birthday was four days away, and I began thinking about how we could celebrate. A small ache had settled in my heart as the distance between us grew. I longed for the days of planting gardens and dreaming of llamas.

The book with its secret pockets and alluring titles was on the back burner for now, shoved under the sofa. Sometimes, in the middle of the day, I would take the rock Chris had put under my pillow and roll it around in my hand, feeling its smooth edges. I had suggested we move on to the next chapter, but Chris said it was too difficult to complete most of the activities while I was prone. The irony was not lost on me. Under normal circumstances, prone would be the ideal position for kindling romance.

I couldn't pinpoint the exact moment it happened, and I couldn't define what we'd lost; I only knew we didn't have it anymore. There was no one to blame. The role of caregiver is a taxing one, and I wasn't exactly oozing sex appeal. *The Ten-Second Seduction* felt like a sham. With my own relationship in embers, how could I possibly provide suggestions to others about firing up theirs?

Maybe I needed to take my own advice. I'd been writing this book about finding and keeping The One. Well, I had found him. Now I had to keep him. I had an hour a day to be in the upright world. I called him up and asked if he would like me to make dinner reservations at our favorite cozy restaurant on the waterfront to celebrate his birthday; we would eat fast. He was all in, excited to get a break and thrilled that even on bed rest, I hadn't forgotten his birthday. Good food, a sip or two of forbidden wine, and time when Chris and I didn't have to talk about work, renovations, or bed rest. I requested a window table, where we could glimpse the Hudson River and have a nice view of the quaint shop-lined street. I googled the menu, planning my entire meal in advance, suffering over the choice between buffalo mozzarella or the frisée and endive salad.

That afternoon, feeling lighter because I finally had some-thing fun to look forward to, I picked up the ringing phone to hear Nadine's voice on the other end.

"Mitchell and I are coming up!" my mother-in-law chimed through the line. I wasn't sure if she was asking me or telling me, but one thing was certain: their visit meant that I was going to have to start wearing clothes again. It had been so hot, I spent most of the time stripped down to my maternity bra and a pair of cotton shorts. "We want to celebrate Chris's birthday," she continued.

I wondered if she was coming to see me, too. My mother-in-law and I were still working out our relationship. We both wanted to be close, but we just couldn't quite fit the puzzle pieces together. When I talked to Chris about it, he told me that it had been hard for her to allow another woman to come between them. She wanted him to have the world, to get mar-ried and have a family, but it also hurt. When Chris and I were first dating, she tried to break us up by telling him I was only dating him for his house—yes, the one with the car frame holding up the basement ceiling, the one with jalousie windows and ancient wiring, not to mention the vomit-brown sofas from 1974. I'd laughed. The last thing I cared about was where I lived; it was whom I lived with and his ability to kill vermin that mattered.

I'd almost forgotten that I was still holding the phone to my ear, until she said, "I'm bringing my pottery. I've been taking private lessons to learn how to glue back together shards of broken antique vessels. I'll show you all the pieces."

I panicked. This was the first time they would be visiting since I began bed resting. Would the house be clean enough for her? How would I keep her and Mitchell entertained from bed? What if they got hungry? What if they needed a towel or soap? Who was going to change the guest room sheets before they got here? All these questions whirled around in my head, but only one word came out of my mouth.

"Okay," I said.

A low guttural howl from deep within Satchie Red's soul marked the arrival of my in-laws two days later. My mother-in-law called from the doorway, "Hello-o-o! Anybody home?" Satchie Red was so excited to see Nadine, purveyor of treats and decadent table food, that her hindquarters wagged along with her tail. Nadine dropped her Louis Vuitton carryall in the family room and dabbed at the beads of sweat on her moist forehead with a neatly folded tissue. She called to her husband, "Mitchell, please get the rest of the bags." She grabbed her hip and groaned, "Oof, my sciatica is acting up. I brought a full cooler from Whole Foods. Is Chris home?"

"Hello. Good to see you." I sat up, running my hands over my boobs to make sure I was wearing a shirt and bra. "Chris is at work," I continued. I thanked her for the cooler. Food really is the universal sign of love. Nadine and I didn't have the closest relationship, but by bringing food, like my mother, she was letting us know she loved us without having to come out and say it.

"Can you get me an ice pack?" she said, plunking down in the pink-and-blue-striped chair, her half-blind, fully deaf cocker spaniel Gracie settling in at her feet.

"Um. They're in the freezer." The hostess in me wanted to jump up to get her an ice pack *and* make her lasagna. I was taught that a good Jewish wife feeds and caters to anyone who walks through her door. "I know how you feel, I have both hip dysplasia and sciatica."

"Aileen, dear, I remember being pregnant. This is nothing like that. This," she closed her eyes and rubbed her hip, "is much worse." She squirmed in the chair, choosing not to get up for an ice pack.

An awkward and silent interlude followed.

I averted my eyes, looking around the room, trying to find new patterns in the knotty pine. Mitchell headed to the guest room with the *Wall Street Journal* tucked under his arm, mumbling something about checking his stocks. Nadine reached into her bag and pulled out a medium-sized Tiffany box. She took such care opening the box, I thought the Hope Diamond must be inside. After painstakingly unfolding the thin white crepe paper, she presented four shards of pottery, holding one up for closer inspection. "This is from eighteenth-century China. The vase is worth a few thousand dollars. But it's broken. I bought it like this on eBay and now I'm going to piece it back together and sell it." Not exactly what I had in mind. She struggled out of the chair and continued taking boxes full of shards out of her bag, arranging them on the table. Next she took out glue, paints, and brushes, in effect creating her very own restoration station right in the middle of the family room.

The following morning, we went to a nearby restaurant for Chris's birthday brunch. Or I thought it was his birthday brunch, but suddenly we were discussing plans for Chris's actual birth date—the day for which I had planned our romantic evening. "We'll all go out to dinner," Nadine announced, not asking anyone else's thoughts on the subject.

I looked at Chris, hoping he would explain that there was a misunderstanding, that we already had dinner plans. I took a bite of my omelet and waited.

"We can invite your aunt and uncle," she continued.

I willed Chris to speak up and kicked him under the table, hard, but he sat next to me nodding along.

"You know, I think we should invite their kids, too," Nadine said, unstoppable.

Was this really happening?

"Sounds good," Chris said as he chewed a forkful of French toast.

I had to brace myself on the edge of the table so I wouldn't keel over. Chris had been so happy when I told him I had made plans. I wanted to hold on to that happiness, revel in it. We needed to find a way to reconnect. The romantic dinner I had been planning would probably be the last and only one before the baby arrived. I had put so much hope into that evening, banking on it to infuse a bit of tenderness back into our marriage.

I knew nothing I wanted to say would come out diplomatically, so I remained silent. It was only when we were alone that Chris sensed something was wrong.

"I was looking forward to spending time with you," I admitted.

"It'll be fine."

"I know your mother has good intentions, but by making this party so big, I can't go."

"It'll work out."

"How is it going to work out if you don't tell her?"

"What's the big deal, Aileen?"

"I made reservations for two. We had plans. If you prefer a bigger party, that's okay, but couldn't we at least discuss it first?" And then in the silence, I whispered, "I thought it would be special, you know, being with you."

"I'm not going to insult my mother."

"Just your wife?"

But he had already walked away and I was left stewing in my bed, like a big old roast. I wished he would have acknowledged my disappointment, but more than that, I had hoped he had been looking forward to that evening as much as I had been. I looked down at my swollen belly, big and pointy, and wondered if my kid was a cone head. "Well at least *you're* spending time with me. You have no choice."

When I awoke in the morning, Chris had already gone to work and Nadine was on the phone inviting friends who summered in the Valley to what was now being called a "Birthday Bash." If Chris hadn't cared to approach his mother about all this party planning, it certainly wasn't my place. She and I spent the rest of the morning watching the home improvement channel. I wondered if she had an inkling of my hurt feelings; if no one had mentioned our plans, I couldn't blame her for wanting to celebrate her son's birthday. We chatted about fixing up the farmhouse, updating the kitchen, and the possibility of painting the knotty pine to brighten the family room.

Early afternoon Chris came home unexpectedly. "Just had to get some tools from the garage. How's everyone doing here?"

"Your mother and I are redecorating the family room. What do you think of painting this paneling?"

"Are you kidding me? Pop put that up."

"It's awful," Nadine argued.

"We'll talk about it later," Chris said, which meant we would absolutely not talk about it ever.

"Chris, Mitchell and I are going to that new café for lunch. Would you like to come along?"

"We are?" Mitchell asked to no one in particular.

"Sure. That'd be great," Chris answered.

"Oh," I said, more to myself than anyone else. He never took lunch.

"I'll meet you guys there in fifteen minutes," Chris called to his mother before closing the door behind him.

My brain knew it was perfectly reasonable for Chris to want to spend time with his mother. But my heart wondered why he didn't want to spend time with me. Did he even think about me anymore? Not the pregnant, bed-resting me—I knew he was concerned about her—the real me. The girl underneath this giant belly. The one he'd planned his life with, traveled to Costa Rica with, the one that smelled like a peach and had a great smile. Maybe he hadn't seen her in a while, but she was still there, waiting.

A strong stench wafted across the family room. Satchie Red was farting. Really farting. Like run-for-your-life kind of farting. That morning I had caught her eating Gracie's kibble, and we were now experiencing the explosive effects.

"Phew! That's horrible. I'll take Satchie Red out before we go," Nadine said, gathering her purse. "Mitchell, honey, please get Satchie's collar."

"I'll do it, don't worry," I said.

As part of my upright hour, I'd started taking out Satchie Red each day for a few minutes to get some much-needed circulation to my legs and fresh air to my lungs. In these moments I could pretend that I was a normal person walking her dog. It was a simple joy I'd come to cherish.

"Mitchell, are you getting the collar?" she called out. I wasn't moving fast enough. She was trying to be helpful. For her, and every other non-bed-resting person, it would seem she was doing me a favor.

"Please, just go. I've got it," I said. I was trying to hold on to something. Everything was slipping out of my control. I had become invisible.

"All right," she said, with a slight twitch in her eye that told me it was anything but all right. "Mitchell, let's go."

When I heard their car drive away, I made my way up and out at a sloth's pace. Standing in the middle of our field while Satchie Red did her business, I saw the sun's afternoon rays glistening against the windows of the Mohonk Mountain House. I closed my eyes, listening to cardinals twittering around the bird feeder that Pop had rigged in the middle of the currant patch. The breeze caressed my skin, cooling the perspiration on my brow. The overgrown grass bending beneath my sandaled feet cushioned my soles. I stood up taller. Lighter.

A sharp tug jerked my arm. Satchie Red was gone. She tore through the yard, chasing a doe. For the love of God! What was her plan if she caught it? And then it occurred to me, she was leaving. The dog was leaving, just like everyone else had that day. I couldn't lose Satchie Red. But I couldn't chase her. I called after her, but it was no use.

With one hand on each side of my lower back, I made my way around the perimeter of the house. After five minutes I was forced to stop, my hips grinding painfully. I backed myself down onto the front steps, overgrown with weeds, and leaned on my elbows. "Satchieeeee." I was met with only the chatter of two yellow finches perched in the blue spruce.

How was I going to take care of a real live baby if I couldn't even take care of my dog? Everything I set out to accomplish was a failure: my marriage, my pregnancy, *The Ten-Second Seduction*, and now I had failed my dog. I looked down at my belly. "I will not fail you. Please, just stay in there. Be healthy." I said it to my baby. I said it to myself. I said it to God.

"You're not a failure. Stop saying that already. Don't be so dramatic." It was my father's voice.

"I didn't expect this to be so hard."

"It only gets worse, my dear."

"Thanks."

"There's nothing wrong with failure. How else can you measure your success?"

I sat with his words.

And then, twenty minutes later, there Satchie Red was, her brown nose poking out between wild forsythia as she emerged from the forest. In a moment she was standing in front of me, panting with her purple tongue hanging out the side of her mouth. She grinned from one pointy ear to the other with an expression that let me know that whatever I was going to do to her, it had been worth it. I grabbed her by the scruff of her wrinkly neck, pulling her toward me, dried tears and hair plastered to my face, and then I buried my head in her shoulder. I could have admonished her, but to what end? In truth, I wished I could be as free as she'd been. Instead of shying away like I had expected, she stood there aloof as ever and let me love her.

We walked back into the house, Satchie Red's eyes glazed over with a faraway look, reliving her recent adventure. In the family room, about to get back onto the sofa bed, I stopped. "No," I said, shaking my head. I had been alone in that bed for too damn long. I straightened my shoulders. And then began searching the house for my car keys, thankful that by whatever means, both the Honda and the Pathfinder were finally back in our possession. Once I found the keys, I grabbed a purse out of the closet, jammed in my wallet, three tissues, and my cell phone. As I put my hand on the kitchen doorknob to leave, I hesitated. I hadn't even checked myself in the mirror. My hair was a tangled nest. My face naked. I turned back, rummaging through the bottom of my bag until I found an old tube of red lip gloss. I picked the lint off the top, squirted out a dab, applied it, smacked my lips together, and slammed the door behind me.

Situated in the Honda, I froze. How did this thing work again? Driving would never be intuitive for me. I turned the key in the ignition and floored it. Wrong way. Brake! Reverse.

I rolled my eyes and looked up to heaven. Shifting gears, I took a deep breath and then exhaled. I had nowhere to go. I wasn't driving myself to the city, especially since I could barely make it out of the driveway. I hadn't thought this through. And then I remembered. There was only one safe haven for me in the Valley.

Jackie came running out as I pulled into her driveway. "Get in here! On my couch, now!" She grabbed my arm, helping me from the car. Her hair was wet, and I could see gray roots peeking through the red. She was in a bathrobe, and from her lips dangled a cigarette, which she now threw to the ground and stomped out. "Sit. Tea? I'm getting dressed." She shuffled me inside.

"I'm done, Jackie," I said.

"You're not done. You're almost done. Sit down."

She left me standing in her living room. The floors were a shiny walnut and every piece of baroque furniture had been carefully chosen for the space it occupied. When I maneuvered myself onto her massive microfiber sofa, the floral cushions swallowed me whole. I didn't know if I'd ever be able to get up again. "I'm over this bed-rest thing," I said when she returned.

"Yadda, yadda, yadda. Relax," she responded, raising her hand.

I glanced down at the shirt I was wearing. The words "Pregnant Diva" were emblazoned in elegant pink penmanship across the front of it. Directly on top of the words was a glittery crown. And right in the middle of it all was a giant yellow stain. Behold the glamour.

For the next hour I sipped tea while Jackie gave me a comprehensive overview of various family members currently on her hit list, until my cell phone rang. It was Chris. I didn't pick up. There were so many times he hadn't answered my calls, was too busy or otherwise occupied. Then Jackie's phone rang. Of course, where else would I be? I had all of one friend in upstate New York. She handed me the phone.

"What are you doing there? I was really worried," he said.

"I'm not coming home."

"What are you talking about?" he asked. He hadn't even realized. He didn't see me for who I was anymore or what I needed in this relationship. How could hc not have the slightest clue?

"I can't do this anymore." Saying it out loud made it real.

"What are you talking about?"

"I'm not coming home," I said again.

"You can't live at Jackie's house."

"I can't live at yours either."

"Ours," he said.

"It's never been mine."

"Come home."

I hung up the phone, and still holding the receiver, I wondered, what now? I listened for my father's voice. But he wasn't there.

"You can stay as long as you like, but you're going to have to face him eventually," Jackie said as she refilled my teacup.

I took a few more sips and then struggled to pull myself up off the sofa and made my way to the bathroom. When I came back, just as I was about to sit down again, I looked toward the door. It was getting late in the afternoon. If I sat down on that sofa again, I'd have to wait until I gave birth before I could find the energy to get back up. I thanked Jackie for her hospitality and with her help got back in my car, this time saying the word "reverse" out loud like David Hasselhoff in *Knight Rider*, just to make sure the car and I understood each other.

My anxiety went into overdrive as I got closer to home. My hands gripped the steering wheel; my head throbbed. Would I walk in there and have to defend myself to Chris and his family? Would they think I was irrational? I felt irrational. I might walk into the house a married woman and leave a single mother.

I stood in the doorway. Chris and I were face-to-face. I had to suck in my lower lip to keep from spewing the barrage of words that had been bottled up for the last fourteen weeks. I waited for him to speak.

"This isn't working, Aileen," he said.

"You're never around. A relationship can't work if one partner isn't there."

"I don't think you understand—I'm trying to hold it all together."

I looked at his face. I loved this man. But here we were. Everything he said was true, but I didn't care. "And how's that going for you?" I retorted.

"What's that supposed to mean?" His tone was louder and more menacing than I'd ever heard.

I wanted him to see me, really see me right now in this moment, needing love, without having to ask for it. I paused, waiting as Mitchell walked through the room toward the master suite with a can of opened paint. "Did you ever consider that I'm trying to hold it together, too? Your priorities are in the wrong place. Family. What about your family?"

Chris turned and began walking away.

"You can't deal with this, can you? That's why you're never here." With every word I said, I was forging a deeper wedge between us.

He turned to me. "I need to work, Aileen."

"I need a husband, Chris."

His ears flamed red, his eyes narrowed. His back ramrod straight and his head jutting out from his neck, hands clenching and unclenching. Is this what he looked like before he went in for the kill? I had never seen him fight.

Now I could hear my father's voice: "Cool it, Kabeen."

"I need space," Chris said, drawing out each word.

"You can have all the space you want. I'm going home," I roared back, holding my belly.

"This is your home, Aileen," he yelled, matching my tone.

"No. This has never been my home. I don't belong here." I didn't know if I belonged anywhere.

"Fine, go if you want to." He threw up his hands in exasperation, turning away from me.

My heart beat so fast that I felt my blood rushing to my ears. I followed him through the house, as we both spilled forth months of frustration. Mitchell walked by with a half-painted baseboard.

I wanted Chris to tell me to stay. I wanted him to turn around and take me in his arms and tell me it had all been a terrible misunderstanding. I needed just one reason not to leave. I needed to know that we weren't together out of obligation, that he still loved me the same way he had two years ago when we were standing beneath the stars and making plans for our future.

I made my way to the closet where I struggled to pull out our huge suitcases, the tags from Costa Rica still attached. "I need my suitcase. Can you please get me my suitcase?"

"Fine! Take it." He pulled out the small one.

"Not that one. I want the big red one. The nice one." He jammed the smaller one back in the closet and pulled the bigger one out above it.

I called my mother. "You can't take the bus. You'll go into labor," she hollered through the phone.

"I don't care." I emptied my drawers into the suitcase, looking for my toiletries, stopping only to catch my breath.

"My grandchild will not be born on a smelly bus with gum stuck to the floor. Do you understand me? Do you want a bus driver to deliver your baby? I have to go. I'll call you right back."

Two minutes later the phone rang again. "Don't take the bus, but if you want to take the bus, I'm sure it will be fine. But don't take the bus," my brother Mark said.

"I'll drive you to the bus stop, Aileen. Just tell me when you're ready," Chris spat out from the other end of the room where he was pacing. I hung up the phone with my brother and turned to Chris, his face hardened, his lips a grim straight line.

"So, is this over?" I said. Mitchell walked by again, this time with a hammer and a set of nails.

"I don't know. I don't know anything anymore." His words hung thick in the space between us. My throat was dry, and it hurt to swallow. We glared at each other, daring the other to speak first. Maybe this whole marriage was a mistake. Or maybe it was just a really bad fight. I couldn't tell. I pictured myself getting on the bus and never looking back, raising my baby as a single mother in Brooklyn. My head was pounding with uncertainty.

The doorbell rang, and I was glad for the small reprieve. I could see out the window that it was Charlie Chaplin with yet another air conditioner. Chris jumped at the opportunity to extricate himself, and I sat on the bed trying to slow my racing heart.

The last time I had run away from home I was fifteen. I had packed my clothes and headed to the house of a friend whose mother didn't ask questions. Life on the run wasn't all it was cracked up to be, so on the fourth day, when my parents came to find me at school, I went willingly. Once home, my mother told me to stay in my room and said that I'd be lucky if I ever saw the light of day again. "Aren't you at least proud that I went to school? How many runaways do you know who go to school?" I asked.

"That's the only reason you're still breathing right now." Later I found out that she had called the school each day to make sure I was showing up, so she knew I was still alive. She slammed the bedroom door behind her then left for work. At 3:00 that afternoon I emerged from my room to find my father on the couch.

"Can I go out?" I asked, knowing that I was taking my life into my own hands.

"You had your mother worried sick," he said.

"And you?"

"I know you can take care of yourself."

"Can I go?"

"The next time you pull this crap, you're dead. You hear me?"

I nodded.

"Get out of here."

As I turned to leave, I paused. "Wait, what just happened?" Even I knew I had crossed a line, that I should be locked in my room and fed through a slot in the door until I was twenty-one, but instead, my father had chosen leniency. He still trusted me to make good decisions, even though I had been so stupid. He chose to set me free to make my own mistakes. The more I thought about it, the more I understood. He'd been doing this my whole life.

Calmer now, it dawned on me that I physically couldn't make the trip to Brooklyn. Once, I had climbed a mountain in high heels, and now I couldn't even lift my own suitcase. I couldn't stand and wait for the bus. I couldn't even sit upright for the two hours it would take to get there. I couldn't go up or down all those subway steps to catch the Q train. The same emotions were running through my body now as when I ran away all those years ago—anger, loneliness, sadness. But my father had trusted me to make good decisions, and I needed to do that now, not only for myself but for my baby and for my marriage.

Chris placed the air conditioner on the floor by the bed and began opening it. I saw it right away, the same dent as the last one. They must be leaving the factory like that. There was no relief of any kind. "I can't handle any of this," he said.

"You mean you can't handle me."

"Do you want a ride to the bus? If not, I'm going back to work."

"I can't make it on the bus. I have no choice. I have to stay for now." I suppressed a sob, though I wasn't sure if it was because I couldn't leave, or because I hadn't been asked to stay.

I buried my face in my pillow. And then I heard the side door slam shut.

When I awoke, I approached Nadine, who had been hiding out in the family room. At the very least, I had not been a good hostess, and at the most, I had outright offended her. "I'm sorry," I offered.

"That's fine," she said.

I understood that we weren't going to have any kind of heart-to-heart. There would be no crying or hugging. That simply wasn't how things were done in this family.

Chris came home that evening, and they went out for dinner without me. This time they asked if I wanted to join them, but everyone was visibly relieved when I declined. Nadine said that she and Mitchell would be leaving in the morning. It was implied but not stated: there would be no party.

The next afternoon I rifled through all the maternity clothes that I'd never had a chance to wear. I had gotten my wish, but it had been a steep price to pay and there was no victory here. Chris and I hadn't resolved anything, but I had hoped to salvage his birthday celebration. I told him I was sorry about how things had unfolded and that I still wanted to take him out to dinner. He agreed, so here I was pulling out a pair of black flared pants and a flowing white bohemian blouse that tied at the top, showing just a hint of cleavage.

Once we were down by the river, I was so giddy to be dressed up and out in public that I playfully pulled Chris along the sidewalk and into the restaurant, but he rolled his eyes and told me to slow down, mistaking my enthusiasm for impatience. I longed for us to reconnect, to enjoy this moment, for him to understand that this was the first time I had done something exciting in months, but he had put up a wall, and I wasn't sure I could breach it.

The table near the window was small and round and I felt twice as big. By the end of the first course, I had a balsamic vinaigrette stain on my right boob. Chris looked at me as I blotted. "Keepin' it classy," I joked. He cracked a smile. Buffalo mozzarella, gazpacho, and a small portion of ravioli tempered the space between us. I gazed out the window at two young parents holding hands, a toddler on the man's shoulders, tapping his father's head. Would we ever be those people?

At home we both fell into bed, exhausted from the tight grip of silence between us. I knew if I waited a moment longer, I'd hear his breathing deepen as he fell into a fitful sleep.

I turned to face him. "I have to leave." I didn't say for how long or if I was coming back, and he didn't ask.

"Okay," he replied, staring at the ceiling. "I'll drive you down." And then he rolled over and went to sleep.

27 | Take Me Home

Weeks 32–33

When I woke in the morning, I began packing, not sure what to bring or how long I would be gone. I rummaged around for an extra belly-support band, thinking duct tape would work better. Thrusting myself into the back of the closet and holding on to a pair of hanging jeans for support, I found a black maternity dress with a small ruffle on the right shoulder. I had hardly worn any maternity couture, but now I was heading back to see old friends who would appreciate the effort. I found my makeup case, checking for mascara. I hesitated, then thought, *Fuck it, the tiara's coming, too.* Dress, mascara, tiara. I was ready. The rock Chris had given me was on the night table. I picked it up and held it to my heart before setting it back down again.

That afternoon Chris loaded the car and I reclined my seat all the way back. Satchie Red hopped in behind me. I looked over at my husband's hand, willing him to place it on my lap the way he used to, but he kept his eyes on the road, lost in thought. I fiddled with the radio, and for the next few hours looked out the passenger window, watching as the tree-lined Palisades Parkway turned into concrete buildings. By the time we reached the West Side Highway, the wind on my face hit me hard, and some stale, sleeping part of me began to awaken. Chris cursed at a driver in the left lane trying to cut him off as the downtown traffic around Chelsea Piers slowed to a crawl, but I was lost in my own world, admiring the strong bodies of the men and women sprinting along the promenade. I longed to feel as light and free as their wide strides made them look.

We inched through the Battery Tunnel and onto the BQE, and when I saw the old men playing chess at the stone tables along Ocean Parkway, the tension I had been carrying in my shoulders for the past months began to dissipate. As we made a left onto Avenue J, the Jewish capital of South Brooklyn, I raised the back of my seat. Chris's hands tightened around the steering wheel with each double-parked minivan he circumnavigated. Orthodox women dressed in ankle-length black skirts and white shirts that covered their wrists, surrounded by gaggles of children, were pushing carts and strollers full of groceries. The line was down the block for Di Faro's legendary five-dollar-a-slice pizza, which I'd never tried. (Who has time to stand in line for pizza?) Isaac's Bakery was getting a delivery, and the truck was blocking one whole lane. By the time we pulled onto my mother's street, Chris was speeding and slamming on the brakes, speeding and slamming. I was quiet. We were almost there. We found parking a block away and walked to my mother's apartment in silence, Chris carrying my suitcase.

Spare key in the door, the smell of other people's dinner seeping through the walls, an amalgamation of roasts, spices, and Chinese takeout. I found a note on the counter saying food was in the fridge, signed with a stick figure of my mother holding a frying pan. I scanned the living room, catching my eye on the mahogany breakfront. Resting on a shelf was a photo of my father holding up a filled-to-the-brim wineglass at Les Deux Magots in Paris and a Matchbox Ferrari I bought him one Valentine's Day. This was not the place where I grew up, but my mother, the pink velvet rocking chair, the aroma of sautéed onions and olive oil in the kitchen . . . It still felt like home.

I backed myself onto the sofa, overcome with relief, breathing in the entire city through the open window. It almost felt like I hadn't been getting enough oxygen for the last few months, and now, suddenly, I was flooded with it. I listened to the familiar buzz of air conditioners and the muffled booms of televisions. A child cried in the alley, a dog barked, construction workers sawed into metal; it all happened beneath my mother's window. There was a steady hum, a hustling of people in the streets below living and laughing, and though I couldn't join them, I could be near them, and this loud chatter soothed me. Chris and I made a quick meal of my mother's leftovers, and then he stood up to leave.

"I have to head back."

"Okay."

He planted a small peck on my forehead before reaching for the doorknob.

I knelt down to give the dog a hug, but she wriggled out of my reach and followed Chris down the hall. There was no fanfare in their goodbye.

The next morning I woke up to construction workers banging on the roof above my mother's sixth-floor apartment and made my way over to the sofa, delighted to find that she had hundreds of cable channels. I was glued to the screen, watching shows about babies, new mothers, and birth—an unexplored television genre! Whereas previously I wanted nothing to do with anything pregnancy-related, now I was hooked. The best part was, there was a marathon of pregnancy-gone-wrong shows, but after the first few episodes, I caught on to the fact that they always turned out just fine. What more could a woman in the final weeks of bed rest ask for? I was four hours into shows about women who had no idea they were pregnant and were now giving birth in random places, when my mother joined me.

"I want to talk about my funeral," she said.

"Right now?"

"I have insurance."

"Great, we're all set then." A woman was giving birth in a gas station, screaming at the attendant to call an ambulance. She had just gotten out of the car, holding her stomach, saying that she thought something was wrong. Suddenly, her water broke, right next to the squeegees. There was no way she was going to make it to the hospital.

"I also have papers," my mother said.

"You have papers?" I was riveted to the screen.

"You'll have to shred them."

I turned to her now. "Are they top-secret papers?"

"I want you to use the same funeral home that we used for your father."

"Are you planning to die today? Because if not, I'd really like to see if this lady gives birth in the gas station. Don't push. Don't push. Hold on. Help is on the way," I called to the TV.

"I'm etching your initials into the furniture that you are going to inherit. This way you don't fight over it with your brother."

"Ma, I don't want your furniture."

"You don't want my furniture? What about your father's armoire?"

"Look, look," I said, pointing at the television, "the baby is coming. Push it back in!"

"Why are you watching this?"

"You're right, Ma," I said. "I'd much rather talk about death and armoires. Etch Mark's initials on all the furniture."

"You just stabbed me in the heart." She grabbed her chest and threw herself backward, then continued, "I wrote down exactly what I want to happen and how I want to be buried. And I don't want my tombstone sinking like your father's. I swear when I visit the cemetery, his plot smells like cigarette smoke."

Then we spent the next fifteen minutes deciding on what New York Jews refer to as *appetizing* for my mother's funeral, which is basically any kind of fish you can put on a bagel—

lox (nova, because belly is too salty), sable (make sure it's filleted), and whitefish salad (taste it so you know it's fresh). Oh, and tuna fish (you can make it yourself because it's just as good as store-bought).

Just when I thought my eyeballs would roll into the back of my head, my friends began arriving for visits. Most had called and emailed while I was on bed rest, but now I was finally seeing them in person. My friend Stella, whom I had met at Cunningham Junior High, bustled in with a big bouquet and shopping bags from Lord & Taylor that weren't for me but filled with skimpy dresses for a wedding she was attending that weekend. We gossiped about boys from our high school, and my mom pulled out my old motorcycle jacket and sweet sixteen pictures just for fun. As Stella was leaving, my friend Laura stopped in. Every morning during college we had met on the steps of the quad to drink coffee and judge our classmates. Now she told me stories of her house renovations and the challenges of teaching underserved kids. As the day wore on, I noticed myself slipping back into my Brooklyn accent and dropping that exhausting letter R. Upstate people always asked me to "talk Brooklyn" to them, as though I were a sideshow distraction, so I had worked hard to hide it. Here, I was just like everybody else. My friends and I discussed everything *except* my pregnancy. To these people, being pregnant was only a small and temporary part of who I was. And because of this, the depression that I had felt so keenly in the early days of bed rest abated until it was just a shadow in the background.

My mother and I fell into a routine. When she came home from work and the temperature dropped from ninety-five to eighty-nine degrees, we would go for a short outing on Avenue J. We often bumped into her friends, women who had full disciplinary authority over me as a kid, and they would joke, "Who gave you permission to be up and about?" In this neighborhood, people were watching out for me.

Growing up, we had been a close-knit community with houses right next to one another; nothing was private and everyone could hear each other's conversations and fights, both our *simchas* and our *shandas*. These women had fed me, yelled at me, and sprayed antiseptic on my naked *tuchus* when I sat on a bee at age three. The kids played handball in the alley and slid down the tops of cellar doors until the sun went down, while our mothers traded recipes and our fathers drank Heinekens on the back steps. As a curly-headed kid who'd never been farther than Long Island and spent most of her time collecting stickers and riding her floral banana-seat bicycle up and down the sidewalk, I had always felt secure around these people.

Once back at the apartment, I would wait for Chris to call, never sure what to say or if he even wanted to speak to me. On most nights the phone would ring after 9:00 p.m., and when I picked up, I could hear the television blaring in the background. I talked to him about my day, told him about the people I had seen, and he responded monosyllabically. He said his days were busy, that he was fine but tired, and after a few minutes of silence, I would tell him it was time for me to get to bed.

One evening, my mother came home from work saying her friend Zahava was on her way over for coffee and rugelach. When I was four, Zahava and her family had moved in downstairs from us on East Eighteenth Street. On the day of their arrival, my brother and I stood on the stoop, a suspicious two-person welcome wagon, sizing them up, trying to decide: friend or foe? Zahava smiled as she passed, and her Israeli husband, carrying their young son on his hip, stopped to say something to us. We couldn't understand a word of his gruff accent, so we cowered backward, wide-eyed and mute.

A week or two later, as I was sitting on the stoop making pot holders with a loom, Zahava asked if I wanted to go for a walk with her while she pushed her baby in the pram. I hopped off the stoop, leaving both loom and loops strewn on the steps. We were halfway down the block when my mother's shriek rattled the front windows of every house within a half-mile radius. I turned to see her running in our direction. When she finally caught up to us, she let loose a tirade on Zahava for kidnapping her child. I don't know what transpired after that, but they must have worked it out pretty quickly, because Zahava became one of my mother's closest friends.

As my mother was in the kitchen preparing coffee, Zahava sat down next to me. I asked her if she had news of any of my Orthodox friends, and she told me who was having babies and who had made *aliyah*—the act of moving to Israel to elevate oneself in the eyes of God. Part of me wanted to see them, and the other part of me still felt forsaken, now more than ever. I couldn't imagine sharing my current marital problems with Rachel—I didn't want to prove her right, that Chris and I were too different to make our marriage work.

"How's the farm?" she asked, raising a skeptical eyebrow over her wire-framed glasses.

"I think my marriage is in trouble," I said.

"C'mon. I don't believe it. Look, men get scared when a baby is coming." She patted my belly.

"We have so many differences. Our values, our beliefs. Even the way we argue."

"Of course! You come from different backgrounds. You knew that when you married him."

"What if it was a mistake?"

She reached over, taking my hand in both of hers. "Look, you married him. You'll work it out. You think Jewish men are easy to live with? Not a chance. Trust me, Jewish men can be very stubborn."

"All he does is work."

"Same with my husband. For years it was just me raising the kids. It's not a religion thing. It's a man thing. If he didn't work, it would be worse." She pushed my hair back behind my ear. "This is not Brownies; you don't just get to stop showing up to marriage."

"You know about Brownies?"

"The whole neighborhood knew about Brownies. Your mother was very concerned you should quit. How would it look?" She winked.

I shook my head, watching the green leaves flutter on the oak tree outside the living room window. "I don't know how to go back. I don't even know if he wants me back."

"You're not a little girl. You don't get to run away just because it's tough." She got up to shut off a lamp. "Your mother has so many lights on."

"I know. It's like living on the sun."

"What does she have to say about this?"

"I told her Chris was busy with renovations and work, and that it was better for me to be here. She may know something is up, but she's happy she can keep a constant vigil over me and the mealy moths at the same time."

"Your mother knows more than you think. Wait until you have the baby, and then see how you feel. Besides, what are you going to do, live here?" She swept her arm around the room. "You and your mother will kill each other. It's going to work out, cookie. It'll be tough, but it will work out."

My mother came into the room with a tray. "The rugelach might still be frozen. They're a little hard, but they should be okay."

"We don't need the rugelach," I said.

"I defrosted the rugelach, so you have to eat it. Zahava, eat. What can I get you?"

Zahava grabbed a frozen rugelach and took a chomp. "What are you going to do? You have to eat it. She defrosted it." She smiled, shrugging her shoulders as my mother went to retrieve a pot of decaf.

That night I lay in the glow of the streetlamp, unable to sleep. I knew Zahava was right. I couldn't move in with my mother. I wasn't a kid anymore. If I stayed in the city, I'd be committing to raising a child on my own. I thought about my wedding day, how nervous Chris and I were standing at the altar. We'd taken vows, signed a *ketubah*. We'd pledged to be loving friends and partners in marriage, to talk, to listen, and to trust, to cherish each other's uniqueness. The *ketubah* actually said those words: "Cherish each other's uniqueness." I had gotten so caught up in this pregnancy, and Chris had been so distracted by the business, we had stopped seeing each other. We were both cracking under the pressure, but I didn't know if the fissures could be repaired.

My father's old MTA hat was sitting on top of the armoire. He had started working the late shift as a clerk for the Metropolitan Transit Authority during my senior year of high school. One summer day after graduation, I came home and found him on the stoop. I sat down beside him. Since he had started working, he wasn't what I would call happy, but he had a sense of purpose, contentment even, and he and my mother were spending more time together.

"You and Mom are getting along so well. What changed?" I asked.

He thought for a while, taking a drag off his cigarette and then offering the rest to me. I took it from him. "Well, I gave up. I just gave up the fight."

I sort of laughed, surprised at his answer. "How do you mean?"

"I stopped caring who won, who was right—none of that matters. Half the time I didn't even know what we were fighting about. Why die on that hill?" he said.

In the semi-dark of my mother's bedroom, with the buzz of the city humming around me, I heard his voice: "Do you want to die on this hill, Kabeen?"

With less than eight weeks left of my pregnancy, my mother announced that it was time to look at car seats and pack 'n' plays. As one of Brooklyn's foremost authorities on Jewish superstitions, she insisted we wouldn't jinx the health of this baby by making sure he had a safe ride home from the hospital and a place to sleep. I even agreed to let her drive me to the store, which was arguably far more dangerous than violating ancient traditions. My brother had given her his fifteen-year-old Toyota Corolla, which she mostly drove from one side of the street to the other to change spots for alternate side parking. As we pulled up to the big-box baby center, I felt a surge of joy. I was starved for a credit card transaction.

The choices of patterns and colors were overwhelming. I was so flustered, I sought out a sales associate, begging him to help me decide on a pattern that would suit my lifestyle. But then, what *was* my lifestyle? Plaid would look great in a country home. A neutral color would go well in a modern city apartment. This was a high-stakes decision.

"Which do you prefer?" I asked the sales associate. He was a hefty older man with a graying beard, and I got the feeling he was hired for his ability to carry heavy items in and out of the store rather than to pick out color schemes.

"It really depends. What color is your nursery?"

I don't even know where I live right now, how can I possibly answer that?

"Yellow." *I could have a yellow nursery.*

"You can't go wrong with neutral."

"But what if it's for a country house?"

"Then definitely plaid."

I leaned against a row of boxed baby swings, ready to talk this through. He looked like a pretty smart guy; maybe he could tell me where to live. "I don't know if I have a country house," I said.

"You don't know where your house is?" He scanned the store looking for another customer who might need his attention.

My mother came running at me waving a flyer. "Aileen, look, I found a coupon. The plaid one is on sale!" Sold. Spared the task of deciding the fate of my marriage and the living arrangements for my unborn child, the sales associate carried the boxes to the register for me.

Back at the apartment, surrounded by my purchases, I slid into bed. My mother's air conditioner was so old and loud, it felt like I was hiding in the wheel well of a 747. It drowned out every thought I had, except one. *Should I stay or should I go?* I had no idea what Chris was thinking, if he was planning his life without me or just assuming I'd come home. I had been at my mother's for two full weeks. I missed Satchie Red. I had skipped an appointment with Dr. Specialist, and though his pronouncements now held little weight, I wanted to stay the course. But it was hard to leave Brooklyn. And then I remembered standing on that glacier in Alaska staring down into the unknown, looking my fears in the face and at all the risks I had taken. If I didn't go home now, I'd be right back where I started.

I turned to the night table and picked up the picture of my father sitting in his token booth at the Kings Highway train station, probably one of the last pictures ever taken of him. He wore a mischievous grin.

I closed my eyes and listened for his voice. "This is real life, Kabeen. You can't pack a garbage bag full of stuffed animals and run away every time there's a problem. Go home." If I could find empathy for my father after all these years and acknowledge the resentment I hadn't even realized I was carrying with me and then let go of it, if I could finally understand him and love him for the man he really was, and not just the man I *thought* he was, perhaps I needed to do the same for Chris before it was too late.

When we had first wed, our farmhouse with its false foundation had been in danger of collapsing. But we'd secured it with a solid beam. Didn't our marriage deserve the same? Maybe seduction could be accomplished in ten seconds, but making a marriage work takes a lot longer. Maybe even a lifetime.

I picked up the phone and dialed.

"Chris, I'm coming home."

28 | Meltdown

Week 34

The county fair was approaching and Chris had reserved a booth to show off his new line of zero-turn mowers. This meant that he would be working from 8:00 a.m. to midnight all week. He wouldn't have time to pick me up in Brooklyn. Instead, my brother agreed to drive me back upstate and spend a few days.

The temperature was hovering at just above one hundred degrees when Mark pulled up in my mother's old Corolla, which he borrowed so he wouldn't have to drive his colossal minivan. I stood on the curb watching as he loaded the car with the new car seat and the plaid pack 'n' play—items I considered precious cargo. In my hormonal end-of-pregnancy haze, the condition of these items was directly linked to the safety of my child.

Before we could get on the road, my brother had to stop at his kids' Hebrew school for a conference. When we found a place to park, Mark rolled down the car windows partway and shut the car off. "Ready?" he said.

"I'm not leaving this stuff in the car with the windows open."

We were in Park Slope, an upscale neighborhood and very safe, but I still remembered when crime here was rampant. My grandmother had lived in the vicinity for forty years and as children we visited often. Back then, one didn't simply stroll around Park Slope. Hipsters had since slowly infiltrated the area; window boxes replaced graffiti and covered up bullet holes, but old habits die hard. I grew up in a Brooklyn where the safest places were the ones the mafia controlled. When my girlfriends and I walked alone at night, we held our house keys between our fingers so we could stab someone if they tried to push us into an unmarked van. What could possibly make my brother think I would leave valuable merchandise unattended in a car with the windows cracked? It felt like he was asking me to leave my actual baby.

"Get out of the car," Mark said.

"Roll up the windows." I refused to move.

"The car will get too hot if I roll up the windows."

"You grew up in Brooklyn. Why is this suddenly okay?"

"Fine, stay." He walked off and then turned, throwing the car keys in the middle of the sidewalk. I got out and picked them up. I got back in the car, rolled *up* the windows, and sat there until I was so hot my thighs turned red and cleavage sweat soaked through my blouse. I don't know why I stayed in that car. Irrational? Maybe. I was thirty-four weeks pregnant and had been in bed for four months. My marriage was falling apart, and it was a hundred degrees outside. My brain had melted. It never occurred to me to roll down the windows or lock up the car and find a cooler place to sit and wait. My only mission was to keep the car seat and the pack 'n' play safe, as if my life, and my baby's, depended on it.

Tears streamed down my face. A man wearing clogs and a white T-shirt stared as he went by, but when I made eye contact, he pretended not to notice me.

I called Chris in between mournful heaves. "I've been abandoned in Park Slope! He just left me here."

"It's okay."

"I don't even know where the subway is!" I blubbered. I thought about stealing the car and driving it all the way upstate myself. A good plan, but let's face it, I couldn't even drive to the supermarket without a map, let alone figure out where the hell the highway was.

"I'll come get you," Chris said.

"Really?"

"Yeah, really. Just tell me where you are."

No matter the space that had grown between us, I knew then that Chris would not let me die of heatstroke. I had said only a few perfunctory words to him over the last two weeks, but he hadn't hesitated to come to my rescue. The man was going to get in his car and drive two hours to Park Slope right now!

"Give it a few more minutes. See if he comes back," he said.

I turned on the air conditioner, but it was an old car, and only the fan worked. Still wilting, I opened the car door so I could breathe, but there was no breeze. And then I called my mother.

When I told her where I was, the pitch of her response was so high only bats could decipher her words. The worst had happened. I was unsafe, alone on the streets of Brooklyn. In her mind, I was already in the last stages of labor, the baby was falling out, and I was hemorrhaging all over the stoop of a fine nineteenth-century brownstone. She had to find me.

"Just stay put! I'm coming for you!" She hung up, but she hadn't asked me what street I was on. Brooklyn is a pretty big place. It might be a while.

Twenty-five minutes later I saw Mark in the side-view mirror strutting down the street toward the car.

"What's the matter with you?"

"You left me!"

"Why didn't you just lock up the car and come into the synagogue? You know, where it's air-conditioned?" I paused mid-sob. I looked up at him, and then down again at the wet, crumpled tissue in my hand. "That's why I threw the keys at you, stupid. Didn't you realize that?"

"No," I laugh-cried.

"Don't be mad. Come on, let's find a place to eat." We drove around the block to a restaurant and sat in a booth, rolling up the windows and locking the car door, this time without incident. I called Chris to cancel the emergency, but as we were ordering, I had a feeling that I had forgotten something.

"Mom!" I shouted.

"No. I'm Mark. You're Aileen. That's how it works. Mom is that woman with all the energy."

"No. Mom. I called Mom. She's looking for me."

"Right now?"

"She's wandering the streets. We have to find her. She's going to knock your block off."

"What does that even mean, 'knock your block off'?"

"I don't know, but it scared the shit out of me when Dad said it."

"Like, really, the whole block had to suffer because we were idiots?"

I looked out the restaurant window to see a blur of a woman in a long brown flair skirt flying by, pointing a black umbrella straight ahead as though charging. Mark and I looked at each other. She was heading down the avenue toward the synagogue where Mark just had his meeting.

"You'd better do something," I said. "I'm carrying her grand-child. She's not going to touch me."

He raised an eyebrow, pointing to himself. "You want me to go out there?" But he headed toward the door.

"God be with you!" I shouted.

They started arguing, my mother's mouth moving furiously as my brother grinned. She smacked him across his chest with the umbrella. They came back into the restaurant, and if I could have hidden under the table, I would have.

"We worked it out," my brother said, putting his arm around my mother. Then he gave her a big kiss on the cheek.

"You're going to put me in my grave, the two of you. Move over," she said, falling into the seat next to Mark.

"Why do you have an umbrella? There's not a single cloud," I said.

"To hit your brother," she replied, and then we all sat down and had a nice lunch.

29 | The County Fair

Week 34—Four Hours Later

I was home. Despite the morning's misadventures with my brother, I was glad I didn't have to walk through that door alone. Satchie Red greeted me, following me around as I opened the windows to let the country air breathe life into the stuffy house. I checked the fridge: no food. I looked around, resisting the urge to straighten up the place, and then I settled onto the sofa bed while Mark made himself comfortable in the guest bedroom.

A few minutes later the screen door opened and Chris called out. My heart skipped a beat. I had missed him. "How was Brooklyn?" He came over to kiss me on the forehead, but I raised my face to make sure his lips landed on mine.

"Good."

"Glad you're home."

I held his gaze, the space between us thick with uncertainty.

"Me too," I whispered.

"It's quiet around here without you," he said. He stood a moment longer and then went into the kitchen.

"Are you going back to work?"

"Yeah. I just came home to see you for a minute. I'll talk to you later." And then I heard his footsteps retreating as he left. I had wanted him to stay, to ask about the city and have a snack, but my coming back didn't magically erase the emotional distance between us. I had foolishly hoped he'd run into my arms and tell me he couldn't live without me. But that was not the man I married. Even if he did feel that way, he would never allow himself to be that vulnerable. He wanted to move on as if nothing had happened. I, on the other hand, wanted to rip open our hearts and let our raw, unbridled emotions gush forth. I wanted us to ugly-cry and wipe each other's snot from our tear-stained faces until our lips met in a sloppy, passionate kiss leaving us breathless, relieved, and a little embarrassed all at once. I wanted an encounter rivaling Rick and Ilsa's unexpected reunion in *Casablanca*.

In the quiet reverberation left behind with the slam of the door, I put my hand to my chest and held it there. This is why it's called heartache.

"Everything all right?" My brother appeared. "I thought I heard Chris. You're not having a heart attack, are you?"

"I have an idea," I said.

"Historically, when you have an idea, I fear for my life."

"Hey, the Cheerios explosion of '79 was not my fault."

"Actually I was referring to the Cheerios explosion of '81."

"That was *your* idea."

"You wanted breakfast."

"You wanted to clean it up with the kitchen sink sprayer! There were soggy Cheerios under the fridge for months."

"It was the only time Dad called a family meeting," he said.

"Yeah, he gave us a written list of rules."

"I think one of them was, 'No more eating. Ever.'"

"This is nothing like that. I just thought it would be nice to surprise Chris at the fair later tonight, but I need a ride. What do you say? I'll buy you a bloomin' onion and a funnel cake."

"So you are trying to kill me."

"I haven't had a carbohydrate in weeks. Do me a favor and let me buy you an onion."

As we approached the fair, the Ferris wheel spun in a whirl of colors and the line of people waiting to enter the fairgrounds snaked through the parking lot. Chris's booth was nestled between one selling underwear and another selling Jacuzzis. His face brightened when he saw me. He held my arm as I climbed up onto a tractor to sit down, while Mark wandered off to explore, but we only had a minute to talk before he had to turn his attention to prospective customers.

The smell of sizzling pork wafted through the summer night, and the vendor across from us hawked fresh lemonade. I passed the time people-watching. Some families stayed close together while others kept their distance from one another. There were adolescent girls holding hands and older couples who were not.

I counted the pregnant women, too. I hadn't seen any in their natural habitat for months, only in doctors' offices. I saw seven in less than twenty minutes, all smiling and talking. Their hips weren't freezing up, they weren't in any noticeable distress— they were upright and walking. I felt a twinge of jealousy and bit the inside of my cheek. One woman in a canary-yellow blouse with a bump almost as big as mine held the crook of her husband's arm, chatting away. My chats were with the UPS guy. I looked around for Chris. He was talking to someone about stale gasoline. He checked in on me when he could, but mostly I sat by myself waiting for Mark to come back from exploring.

It was a slow march to the exit, the pressure in my uterus bordering on painful. I had overdone it, and now I was paying. I told Mark that seeing all the happy pregnant ladies made me feel like crap.

"You know what Dad would say, right?"

"Yeah, he'd say, 'Here, have my cigarette.'"

"Okay, that's what Dad would say to you. What he'd say to me is, 'Don't always assume other people have it better. Everybody's life sucks.'"

"Profound."

"Dad would be very proud of you, you know, for sticking with this. No one ever really thought of you as the type to commit."

"Is this about Brownies?"

"It's not just Brownies."

"Bed resting doesn't make me a good person."

"No, it just makes you a *different* person."

"Did you think I wouldn't be able to do it?"

"I had my doubts. But deep down I always knew you would."

"So you think somehow I'm different now?"

"Well, I always thought of you as selfish. I admit my opinion is probably skewed because I've put so much effort into hating you, but you put your own needs aside for this baby. And after all the initial feeling sorry for yourself, you began to embrace it. You know what that makes you?"

"Hopeless?"

"No, you idiot. It makes you a mother."

When we arrived home, I got into the sofa bed and my brother brought over a bowl of cashews.

"Those cashews are Chris's only sustenance. Don't eat them all. He'll starve."

My brother shrugged. "Move over," he said, situating himself next to me. Satchie Red jumped down, disappearing into the other room. "Your dog is weird."

"She doesn't like people."

"More room for me." He stretched out his legs. "So, what's up?"

I was still tentative about trusting this "adult" version of our relationship, but what did I have to lose? I confessed every detail of my marriage over the last four months.

"Hmm, I didn't realize it had gotten so out of hand," he said when I was done.

"You asked."

"Let me get some more of Chris's cashews."

I wondered if it had been a mistake to tell him. Perhaps he would use it against me at some later date. He came back, offering me the bowl. "What kind of dog doesn't like people?"

"Did you listen to anything I just said?"

"Yes. And this is what I think. You and Chris never had the opportunity to build a solid foundation. So many things happened so fast. It takes most people a lifetime to go through what you went through in less than two years. His dad dying, moving, buying a rental property, investing in a business, starting a family, possibly losing a baby, being on bed rest. It's like every after-school special jammed into one episode."

"Plus, we have no idea how to communicate with each other."

"True. We yell, we fight, we throw food, and we get over it. Chris probably didn't have that experience as a kid," Mark said.

Not only did Chris not have siblings to throw eggs at, something my brother and I had done on more than one occasion, but he was taught not to make a spectacle. Our family lived for them. The very first time Chris witnessed a disagreement between me and my mother, he was sure I was going to walk out of her life forever. "Don't worry, I'll call her in about twenty minutes," I said. He was mystified. In his family, if two people got into an argument, it could very well mean the end of the relationship.

"Remember how Dad used to yell at us when he was nervous? How we were never allowed to shut the TV off during dinner because he was afraid it would break and he'd miss *All in the Family*? I get the feeling Chris is like that but different," Mark said.

"So you're saying he has anxiety?"

"He just doesn't express it in a way that we can understand. Where Dad would scream and yell, Chris just bottles it up. He's stressed out. You guys are going through some life-changing shit right now," Mark said.

"Dad didn't really like to confide in anyone, and neither does Chris."

"Well, it's no surprise you married a man with similar traits. It probably gives you comfort in some sick, twisted way."

"I wish Dad were here. He always had an answer for everything."

"It's a good thing it was the same answer, no matter the problem."

We turned to each other and both said, "Fuck 'em."

30 | Gumption

Week 35

Adonis is on the deck. He's shirtless. Sweat is glistening off his firm trapezius muscles, ever so slowly gliding down the center of his back. I scribbled the words on a piece of paper to be included in *The Ten-Second Seduction,* and even though I had decided not to send the book out on submission, it was good to get back to my craft. Adonis—or, as he was known to everyone else, Billy—was painting our deck. A former tenant, he was hired in a last-ditch attempt to finish the renovations before the baby's arrival. But Adonis did not make haste. To him, this deck was a masterpiece. *Each upward stroke is a precise and calculated maneuver.*

I looked up from my pen and paper, and it occurred to me that we were paying him by the hour. With two days behind him, he had only put one coat on half the deck.

Note: Fire Adonis.

On the other side of the house, the master suite was even further behind schedule, and I feared my baby would have to sleep in a cardboard box. I had made the executive decision that our washer/dryer needed to be on the same floor as the rest of the house. Until now these appliances had always been in the Basement of Death and Despair, and the washing machine, which had never been connected to the waste line, drained into a huge barrel that had to be emptied halfway through the cycle. Pop thought the suds might ruin the delicate septic. Every time we did a load of laundry, Chris had to haul buckets of dirty water to the far end of the field and dump them. If we timed it incorrectly, the barrel would overflow. Because of this he had insisted we only do washes twice a week. But all bets would be off once the baby arrived. There was zero chance I would be willing to run through the yard with baby-poop water every day.

The man now in charge of accomplishing these renovations was called Wick, and whatever that nickname meant, he was no Adonis. He was more Charles Manson. Chris just showed up with him one day, and I was so desperate to have the work done, I didn't care if he was a convicted killer as long as he could spread grout. Wick was supposed to be laying floor tile in the new laundry room and replacing the front door of the house, which wouldn't open. I had this wild idea that in addition to modern plumbing, it would be nice to have a working front door.

When I got up for a pee break, I waddled over to Wick's work area to check on his progress. "How's it going?" I asked, noticing he had put down a total of four tiles in the last two hours. He stopped what he was doing, squinted at me with dark, shifty eyes, and grunted.

The short gray hairs on his head bristled. I took a few steps back. This guy made Scary Larry look like Peter Pan.

Back on the sofa bed, I watched Adonis through the deck door. He was on a ladder painting the railings. I tried to mind-meld with him, willing him to paint faster. My attempts at thought control had the opposite effect. He stopped, threw down the paintbrush, and sprawled out in the summer sun.

I heard a crash and cursing from the other side of the house. Past experience told me no good could come of this. Sending up silent prayers to God, I shuffled back across the house to find that the four tiles that had been placed were now stacked up against the wall, with mysterious cracks in them. Wick was nowhere to be found. I peeked outside and saw Chris's tools scattered on the lawn. The front door to the house was also on the lawn. In pieces. I heard the sound of a truck starting and the squeal of tires as Wick peeled out of my driveway. Dark clouds formed over the house, and rolling thunder could be heard in the distance. Satchie Red came and stood by my side.

"We're screwed," I said.

She barked twice.

The rain came down hard and fast, and back in the family room, I watched through the window as all of Adonis's work thinned into red streaks and dripped down the white posts on the side of the deck. More money washed away. He was gone, too, no doubt taking off when the rain threatened to ruin his nap. With the front door missing, I wondered how many small animals would take refuge in my house that evening. I placed my palm on my belly, the baby inside growing strong. He'd gained a whole pound as of our last doctor visit, but for each ounce he grew, another piece of our house came down. I did some rough calculations and figured that by the time I reached full term, the house would be reduced to a pile of rubble.

When Adonis reappeared hours later, I broke up with him, saying it wasn't him, it was me. But it was totally him. As I watched his young, strapping body saunter away, I looked down at my maternity clothing; there were stains covering stains. I had nothing to lose. I made my way over to the deck, found a paintbrush, and popped open a can of barn-red paint. I had the brush, I had the paint, and I had the gumption. "It's just me and you, deck," I said.

I studied the paintbrush in my hand, running my fingers over the bristles. Then I surveyed the deck again. The point was for these two objects to meet, but I had no idea how to make that happen with my giant belly in the way. I stirred the viscous red paint, dipped the brush, then bent at the waist as far as I could and swatted the brush onto the deck. It made a messy splotch. That wasn't going to work. I got on my knees but still couldn't quite reach the floor unless I painted myself into a circle. And then I had a brilliant flash of clarity, inventing my now signature move: the Squat-Paint-Shuffle.

There are certain defining moments in a person's life. This was one of them: I had lost my last shred of dignity. I squat-paint-shuffled in twenty-minute intervals, lying down to rest in between, and soon had the whole deck floor painted. There was nothing glamorous about the Squat-Paint-Shuffle, but damn, it felt good. For the first time in months, I was efficient, innovative, and most of all, I felt accomplished. And *that* was sexy.

Wick ignored my calls, and I knew he wasn't coming back. I went over our conversations, trying to figure out if I had done or said something wrong. Maybe it was inappropriate to ask questions like, "How's the floor coming?" or "Can you give me some sort of timeline for this project?"

That evening Chris walked through the doorless doorway. "Why is the front door on the lawn?"

"Because God hates us."

"At least the deck is painted," he said.

"I fired Adonis."

"Adonis?"

"I mean Billy. I painted the deck."

"You did not paint the deck."

"I did."

"No kidding."

"I'm capable of many things."

"I'm beginning to see that." He smiled.

Having both worked on *The Ten-Second Seduction* and painted the deck this week, I was feeling giddy and unstoppable. I told Chris we were going to make a pilgrimage to our local big-box store to order a door, even though I had already far exceeded my allotted upright time for the day. Chris responded by shoving three rapid handfuls of mixed nuts in his mouth.

"I'm glad to see you're diversifying beyond cashews. Do you eat anything besides nuts?" I said.

"It's not like there's a shortage."

This moment, however small, was pivotal. We were on such tender ground that even this little exchange could easily lead to misunderstanding. I paused, then tossed my pillow at him.

He caught it and brought it back to my bed. Then he sat down on the edge and looked out the window. "We live in such a beautiful place," he said.

I examined his profile, his rough, unshaven jaw, the papery skin around his eyes, the soft blond hair that came to a neat line on the back of his neck. "You're working so hard, you don't get to enjoy it anymore."

"I'm not taking care of myself."

"It's been hard for both of us."

"I always thought I'd live on a beach in Brazil and work on my tan."

"I'm sorry it didn't turn out that way."

"No, I'm happy with you. I want to be with you, Aileen." He turned to face me.

"Really? Why? Why do you want to stay?" I didn't know what he could still see in me.

And then he spent the next hour sharing. He told me how he loved coming home at the end of the day just to fall asleep next to me. He told me how he went to work for us, for our family, to build a life together. He loved how I had made the house look nice and how, before bed rest, I cooked big elaborate dinners. He loved hiking the Shawangunk Ridge with me and planning vacations. He'd never had that growing up, but he wanted it now, with me. He enjoyed our outings to small towns like Phoenicia and Hudson, antiquing, trying new restaurants. He told me that there was nothing else in the world that he wanted more than a healthy baby and our little family. He didn't want to be with anyone else. He wanted to be with me.

He chose me. Every day Chris got up, went to work, and chose me. Now it was up to me to choose him right back.

It was humbling to watch this man who rarely spoke more than five words at a stretch sit there and pour his heart out to me. And it seemed he was ready to listen to what I had to say, too. I told him how depressed I had been, especially at the very beginning of bed rest, how no one seemed to notice, how I had been drowning in fear and sorrow. I felt a little better now, though. I talked about Brooklyn and how I never thought I'd end up on a farm in the country. I told him that he worked harder than any person I had ever met, that I respected his dreams and his ambition.

"We've both been so caught up in ourselves, we forgot to check in with each other," I said.

He nodded. "I see where you're coming from."

"Thank you."

"I'm glad we got to talk. Ready to go order a new front door?" He reached his arm out to help me out of bed and to the car.

I wondered if my father, also a man of few words, had ever revealed himself to my mother. During their late-night tête-à-têtes around the kitchen table, when my brother and I were sleeping, my father must have let her into his world, even if it was just for a while. Perhaps those moments were enough to sustain her for a lifetime.

After a heated discussion with various door "experts" at the store, it was determined that the one I had chosen—a red one, with a long narrow glass pane down the middle like a little peep show—would not fit. For that matter, none of the seventy-five other doors they sold would fit the handmade-by-Pop dimensions of our door frame. I waddled to the parking lot in a huff, leaving a trail of verbal bloodshed behind me for all the lucky bastards who had normal houses. I hated those people.

Chris, ever the opponent of air-conditioning, rolled down the car windows, and the breeze helped soothe the tirade running through my head about quirky country houses and how difficult it was to get anything accomplished. As we drove, the setting sun cast a glow over the mountains, streaking the sky with an artist's palette of orange, red, and pale pink. I leaned back and closed my eyes as we cruised down winding roads toward home. No traffic, no noise, just the sweet sound of bullfrogs, cicadas, and crickets awakening to activity.

The sky darkened, and stars popped out one by one. A rustling from the backseat jarred me. I turned my head but could see nothing. Silence. Must have been the wind. I closed my eyes. Then there it was again.

"Do you hear that?" I turned my body around as far as I could, but alas, I had lost my waist and thus my ability to twist.

"I'm sure it's nothing. Close your eyes. Relax."

"What is that?" I said as I tried one more time to turn my body toward the backseat.

"Stop putting your head back there," Chris said as he accelerated the car.

"What in the hell?" I insisted.

"It's nothing. Turn around."

And then something hit me hard in the face. It got tangled in my hair and began fighting its way out.

"Get down! Get down," Chris yelled.

"Down! Down? Down where? I'm eight and a half months pregnant! There is no down!" I shrieked as I tore at my hair.

Chris grabbed the top of my head trying to shove me to the floor as he swerved into the oncoming lane.

"Stop the car. Stop the car!" I said between hyperventilating breaths.

"I can't. There's no shoulder." He swerved back, correcting the wheels just in time.

"Get it out! Get it out!" I flailed my arms. Chris began swatting at my head. "Stop hitting me!"

"I'm trying to get it out!"

About an hour—okay, fifteen seconds—later, Chris pulled into the driveway of a fancy estate, and before he could put the car in park, I had flung open the door and tumbled out. I righted myself, smacking my head and shaking my body, and, as I got to my feet, jumped up and down. Pushing my hair out of my eyes, I paused to catch my breath. It was only then that I saw about thirty people streaming toward me, holding champagne flutes with little strawberries in the bottom of each glass. Their collective mouths were agape. They stopped a safe distance away. An older man in khaki pants and a polo shirt stepped forward.

"Is everything okay?" he asked.

"Something . . . my face . . . hair," was all I could manage.

"Do you need a doctor? Are you in labor?"

"I, I . . ." I was embarrassed. I looked around at the mortified faces of the people standing before me. I had tumbled right into the middle of a wedding. Well, now we'd all have something to talk about for years to come.

"Aileen, take a look," Chris called to me. I inched over to the car and peeked in. There, hanging from the radio on the dashboard, was a black furry bat. The song I had sung to children as an educational leader in AmeriCorps popped into my head about how bats eat bugs, not people. I also taught those children that bats had sonar and that it was a myth that they got tangled in people's hair. I am here to debunk that fallacy.

I turned back to the man still standing there holding his champagne flute. I didn't suppose he was going to offer me any. Chris shooed the bat, but it was so fast, neither of us saw it fly out of the vehicle. It just vanished. "You can get in the car. It's gone now," Chris said.

"How can you be sure?"

"There is no bat here anymore."

"What if I have rabies?"

Chris came over to my side of the car and looked at me. "I think you're okay."

"Well," the nice man said in a calm but perhaps condescending tone. "If you need anything, just let me know. Stay here as long as you like." He and the rest of the guests turned back to the festivities. I had limited options. No subway was going to roll by to take me home. I could handle this. I could get back into that car. I slid into the seat and looked around one more time before slamming the door shut.

"Well that was something," I said.

"You know, you flipped out, but you pulled yourself together. If this had happened a month ago, you'd be having a breakdown right now, yammering about going back to the city. Instead, you got back into the car."

"I guess that's what we call progress."

"You did good. I'm proud of you." He stroked my hair.

"I thought it was the end of days there for a minute."

"Maybe it's just the beginning." And then he put his hand on my knee.

31 | Calypso

When Becca, my massage therapist, came by a few days later, Satchie Red greeted her as usual, planting her nose in Becca's bag in search of edible massage cream. Then she jumped onto the massage table, curling up at my feet.

As Becca kneaded my muscles, I told her how grateful I was to her for being on this journey with me. It was hard to believe that now the journey would soon be ending. While I had spent most of the last five months trying to keep this baby in, something inside me had shifted. I was ready to begin thinking about how this child was going to get out. Becca and I talked about birth plans, but given how the rest of this pregnancy had gone, we agreed that the best birth plan for me was no birth plan—go in for the C-section and let whatever happens, happen. But that's not me. Of course I needed a plan. I needed my plan to have a plan. Becca, who was studying to be a doula, told me that things can change pretty quickly in a hospital setting. "Birthing babies is messy business," she said. "I've seen some women get very upset when things don't go their way. Be open to suggestions."

As she massaged my legs, I considered her advice. I was getting a C-section per Dr. Specialist's suggestion, so I had limited say in how the birth went. But there were things I could do to maintain some control. If I looked at this as more of a spa experience and less as a "cutting you open and ripping a human being out of your body" experience,

248

it might not be so bad. I'd bring snacks, music, scented oils, and foot lotion.

Months ago Chris and I had agreed to hire a doula. This would ensure there would be at least one rational person in the room. We also agreed that our mothers should be at the hospital, and I even wanted my brother there, but only after the baby was outside my body.

When the massage was over, I climbed down from the table and squatted on the floor to stretch my hips, hands in prayer position in front of me.

"You are so ready to birth this baby. You look like a goddess," Becca said. I was taken aback. I had forgotten that giving birth was a spiritual act. "Look at your hair. It's almost down to your elbows when you straighten your curls, and it's so thick. You're glowing."

I bet those sales associates trying to sell me a door the night before didn't think I was glowing, and I'm pretty sure the wedding guests with their champagne flutes thought the only glow I had was that of a wild she-devil. But Becca's words were empowering. I had grown an actual human being inside of me.

Now I just had to schedule when this human being was going to come out. After Becca left, I called Dr. Enchanté's office, but he was on vacation. The nurse told me that she would get back to me with a date. Three days later, as I lounged on our freshly painted deck, she called. "How does September twenty-first sound?" the nurse asked.

I paused. I wasn't sure what she was talking about. "That's my birthday." Was she trying to clarify this for insurance purposes?

"Great, that's when you're having your baby."

"Um, no. No, I'm not."

"That's the date."

"It's my birthday," I repeated.

"And now it's going to be your baby's birthday, too."

"No."

"Most women are thrilled to have a baby on their birthday."

"Yeah, well, I've had a lot of complications with this pregnancy. If something bad happens, I don't want it to be on my birthday."

"Well this is when the doctor can get the OR, and it's not a good idea to go too much longer."

"So you're telling me he can only get the operating room one day a week? No one ever has a C-section on, say, a Monday, or a Wednesday?"

"You'll have to talk to the doctor, but like I said, he's on vacation."

"Maybe you can have him call me because, here's the thing, I'm not showing up for surgery on my birthday." I tried to say this in the nicest possible way. I've heard that if you speak with a smile on your face, it comes through in your voice. I turned the corners of my mouth into an overexaggerated grin.

I was in the home stretch. Everything would probably be okay. But there was still the potential for something to go very wrong during the C-section. If I died, my tombstone would read, "Born September 21, died September 21," and people would point to my grave site and say, "Come look at the girl who died on her very own birthday, how sad!" Or worse (and this was the one that made me stick to my decision), what if I lived and my baby didn't? Every year, for the rest of my life, I would remember that I lost my child on my birthday. I would never celebrate that day again.

Dr. Enchanté called that evening, the sound of Calypso music playing in the background.

"September twenty-first," he said, as if we were in the middle of a conversation.

"That's not going to work."

"Has to."

"It's my birthday. You have to change the day."

There was a long pause and what I'm pretty certain was a slurping sound. Mai tai? Margarita? I couldn't tell. "Okay, I'll see what I can do," he said.

That was as good as a yes as far as I was concerned. I wasn't really that worried. One way or another, this baby was going to come out.

32 | Courage and Cremation

Week 37

"Your uterus has shifted." Dr. Specialist was standing over me, flipping through his notes.

"What does that mean?" I sat up on my elbows and raised an eyebrow, then glanced over at Chris.

"You can have a vaginal birth." He closed my chart and tucked it under his arm.

"What?" I had picked up Chris's habit of pretending I hadn't heard something I couldn't process.

"Your uterus has shifted," he repeated. "Your cervix is no longer obstructed. No need for a C-section." And just like Charlton Heston receiving the Ten Commandments on Mount Sinai, it was decreed.

With the cold gel on my belly starting to get itchy, and agitated by the cheap paper robe sticking to it, I was beginning to feel like this guy maybe didn't get me. I prefer pros and cons, charts, graphs, diagrams, eyewitness testimony.

"I understand this is not a big deal to you, but I could use a few more details."

He looked at his watch, deciding if our three-minute consultation could be pushed to four. He motioned to the screen.

"Your uterus has rotated. The biggest fibroid is no longer blocking your cervix. You can deliver vaginally." With that, he turned toward the door. His work here was done.

"I'm not prepared! I have a C-section already scheduled," I called out.

"Cancel it," he shrugged without turning around.

"Cancel it? Does one simply cancel a C-section? I don't even know how to breathe." I turned to Chris, who had been sitting mute. "Is it too late for Lamaze? Do people still do Lamaze?" The tech cracked a smile as she wiped the goop off my belly. She thought I was joking. I was not joking.

"I guess we'll figure it out," Chris said. "Besides, it will probably mean less time to recuperate afterward."

On the way home, we went over the options I had read about in the baby bibles all those months ago. We could have a home birth, or even a water birth. Babies know how to swim, right? And because the only way I know how to process new information is to talk about it, I called everyone I knew.

From Jackie: "Those bastards. You march right in there and say, 'My name is Aileen Weintraub, I want an epidural.' Don't let them talk you out of it."

From Watson: "Squat. That's what my wife did. Best thing for you."

From the Charlie Chaplin UPS guy, whom I didn't actually call but who came by to deliver a package: "You're going to be great. Don't sweat it. Make sure you get down on all fours. I hear it relieves the pressure."

From my brother Mark: "I bet it's going to hurt. It's very painful. Are you going to take the drugs? You gotta take the drugs."

From my mother: "You know, I had fibroids. I had to get them removed."

Wait. What?

My mother waited until *now* to drop this bombshell?

"You were eleven. I thought you knew."

"How has this not come up this whole time I've been in bed? Why haven't we been talking about this?"

"We're talking about it now."

"What happened?"

"I told you, I got them removed. You were at camp. You came home and you were really upset that I wasn't paying attention to you. I think you threw a chair."

"I remember that! You didn't explain anything to me. I had no idea why you wouldn't get off the sofa. Mark told me you were dying. How could you not tell us? You tell us what you had for lunch three weeks ago." I had never known anyone else who had fibroids, and here my own mother had been avoiding the subject for twenty years.

"I'm sorry. We didn't talk about things like that back then."

"So talk about it now."

"I had a hysterectomy because that's how they removed fibroids at the time, by taking out your whole uterus. It turned out okay. No more heavy periods, no more PMS."

"What about Dad?"

"Dad didn't have fibroids. I don't think men can get them. Can they?"

"No, I meant, where was he?"

"He came to pick me up at the hospital, but as soon as I was home, he left for the rest of the day."

"Did he take care of you?"

"His mother did, and my mother came, too. There were a lot of things your father couldn't handle. We've been over this. He didn't like to be around sick people."

"Yeah, I know. He used to yell at me whenever I threw up."

"Look, I did what I had to do and that was it. I took a few days off from work, and it was fine."

"It was fine? You lost your uterus. How is that fine?"

"There was no one to talk to. You just did. And that was it. You did and you moved on."

All those years she had never discussed her surgery with me and my brother, and my father hadn't helped her through it. I considered my father the easy parent, because mostly he left me alone to do what I wanted, but he was not an easy husband.

My father and mother weren't a team; he wasn't there for her, at least not enough. When I put myself in her shoes, I can't understand why she didn't just leave all of us, but I'm grateful that she stayed, that she kept our family from falling apart.

I'd run out of people to call for birthing advice, so I turned on the television and found Produce Pete talking about broccoli. September was upon us. My mother "just did," and now it was my turn. I looked around at all the pillows and books piled up, the cups and the Ziploc bags filled with snacks. This was the room of a sick person. I wasn't sick. I was having a baby. I didn't have time to be sick.

I hoisted myself off the bed and began putting away all evidence of bed rest: cooler, tray table, the giant mug from my mother-in-law that said "There's Big and Then There's Bubba." Dirty dishes went into the kitchen sink. Tissues and other debris went into the trash. Magazines were neatly stacked on the coffee table. Tiara went on my head. I stripped the sheets from the sofa bed, and as I did so, a surge of energy rose up from my belly into my chest. Somewhere deep within, I was still strong. I braced myself and then lifted up the metal bar at the foot of the bed and tried to push the mattress in and down, angling it into a folded position. I fell on top of it, stood up, and pushed again, harder. For the remainder of this pregnancy, I was going to convalesce like a low-risk pregnant woman nearing full term—sitting on the couch, channel surfing with comfort food and maybe even an occasional glass of wine. I wrestled with the beast as it folded up into itself. Then I sat on it, using the undeniable power of my ass to force it inside its old dusty home. I arranged the cushions on top of it and collapsed in triumph. It was gone.

In clean clothes, with a dab of blush on my cheeks, I met Chris at the door when he arrived home. "I'm done with bed rest. Let's go celebrate." Chris's grin showed his teeth. It was the first time I'd seen him smile in months. It looked awkward and unnatural, like his facial muscles were straining under the new shape his mouth was making. He didn't ask why, or what changed my mind; he just went to the bedroom to put on a fresh shirt.

"Let's go," he said, holding aside the plastic he had put up over the hole that used to be the door.

We headed to a restaurant a few miles from the house.

"I'm nervous about giving birth," I said to Chris after the waitress had placed our sandwiches in front of us.

"It'll work out."

"Labor isn't for the faint of heart. I haven't done any real exercise in months."

"Don't worry."

"If something happens to me, what would you do? I mean with the baby." I took a bite of my tempeh Reuben.

"My mother would help take care of the baby."

"Are you going to eat all those fries?" I asked, throwing diabetic precaution to the wind.

"Help yourself."

"I really want our child to get a college education." I picked a fry off his plate, dipping it in ketchup.

"I don't think colleges accept infants."

"You can get breast milk from a bank."

"Like Ulster Savings?"

"And I want to be cremated."

"You're Jewish. Didn't you tell me it's against the law?" He took a big bite of his turkey sandwich.

"Don't put me in the ground. I'm afraid of the dark."

"You're starting to sound like your mother with her funeral planning."

"Yeah. Well, maybe that's not such a bad thing."

"Okay. Cremation it is. Split an apple crisp for dessert?"

"Don't let my mother talk you out of it. She's not going to like it. Be strong. And keep my ashes. I want to be on the mantle, like your dad, but in a martini shaker, not a beer stein. German chocolate cake?"

"The mantle? Forever? No burial? Strawberry cheesecake?"

"Well, when you die, I thought we could have our ashes mingled together. You know. For eternity. Wouldn't that be nice?"

"Eternity? That's a long time."

"Are we on the same page here?"

"I don't know. How about crème brûlée? We both like crème brûlée."

"I need to know you have a plan."

"Okay, if things don't work out, I will cremate you. And I will find a college for infants."

"Apple crisp sounds perfect."

33 | Jeeps and Rabbits

Week 38

As we watched the birthing video with our doula Anne, who agreed to give us a crash course in vaginal delivery, I had to hold back little bits of puke. It looked more like a murder than a miracle. And why was the lady completely naked? The baby wasn't going to fly out of her breasts. I was not going to be naked. But then, what is fashion protocol for birthing a baby? Maybe I'd repurpose one of my old Shabbat skirts.

After the video, Anne showed us her three-dimensional birthing puzzle, taking apart the uterus and demonstrating how the baby moves through the birth canal. Everything after that was a blur because all I could think was that my husband was never going to have sex with me again.

Chris and I left Anne's office in stunned silence. When we got in the car, he poked me, but I refused to look at him. "You okay?" he asked.

"That was not pretty."

"Yeah, I wasn't expecting that level of detail. Hey, let's take a detour."

"Where are you taking me? I'm feeling kind of queasy."

"Deep breaths. We're going for a ride." He rolled down all the windows.

"Give me a hint."

"Don't you trust me?"

We traveled along winding roads and over an expansive bridge into the next county, every bump making my stomach lurch.

Chris pulled into a deserted parking lot and killed the ignition.

"You have no alibi," I said.

"How do you know?" His mouth formed a devious smile.

We were in a desolate area on the outskirts of Poughkeepsie, surrounded by run-down buildings. Chris tapped the steering wheel, making no move to get out of the car.

"Why are we just sitting here? Didn't you think this through?"

"I have no idea what you're talking about."

"I know you're not super organized, but if you're going to off someone, you should have some sort of plan in mind. You don't just waste all this time thinking about it while I'm sitting right here."

Chris looked at me. Or actually, he looked over my shoulder at the car pulling up alongside us. "Come on! Get out. Look."

A thirtysomething bald man with a round belly, not unlike my own, stood before us.

"What do you think?" Chris said.

"Of the bald guy?" I whispered.

Chris rolled his eyes. "The Jeep."

On second look, the bald guy was indeed standing in front of a Jeep.

"Do you want to test-drive it?" Mr. Bald Man asked Chris.

It took both of them to help me into the backseat. Chris drove the car around the neighborhood and they began to negotiate price. The car was crisp and clean, and it went both forward and backward, something I no longer took for granted.

The negotiations seemed to be going well as we pulled back into the lot, but before I knew what was happening, Chris was calling the whole thing off. They were disagreeing about the inclusion of the stereo system. I tried to intervene, but it was no use. As Chris came around to help me out of the car, he took me aside, telling me it was the principle. None of this really mattered though, because it had been over forty-five minutes since I had last peed. I asked Mr. Bald Man if he knew where the closest bathroom might be.

"Well, that's my office." He motioned to a beige warehouse with tiny windows.

"Do you mind?"

"You don't want to go in there."

"I don't care if you're hanging dead bodies from the ceiling. I've been pregnant for like three years now. You have no idea what it's done to my bladder."

"Mmm. Maybe you can find a gas station."

"Then we have to go right now." I glared at him, trying to penetrate his soul. It was a high-noon standoff. I folded first. "Okay, we'll be in touch." I started climbing into our car.

"Okay. I'll show you the bathroom."

Mr. Bald Man led us around the corner and unlocked a side door to the building. The warehouse was dim, with gray walls and flickering fluorescent lights. A sea of faces looked up from their computer terminals along the wall.

"Down the aisle to the left," Mr. Bald Man said.

I made my way down the long corridor with shelves on one side and stacks of cardboard boxes on the other. A half dozen employees packing and taping these boxes stopped and looked up at me. They seemed startled, like I'd caught them assembling nuclear arms. Why were they staring at me? I looked down at my dress for bodily fluids. It was like they were all in on a secret, waiting for me to understand. On the metal shelves to my left, there were colorful objects wrapped in plastic. Were these medical supplies? I slowed my steps. Curlers? What was the big deal?

No. Oh my God. They were sex toys. Bright neon, purple, magenta, green, all glowing at me. I had never seen so many in one place. There were vibrators, bullets, wands, gels, and enough bondage tape to restrain the New York Giants. I stopped in front of a shelf of rabbits and was just about to pick one up when one of the people behind me coughed. I drew my hand back and continued toward the bathroom. That was the closest I'd come to having sex in almost five months.

"Now you see why I didn't think this was such a good idea?" Mr. Bald Man said when I met him and Chris back by the door.

"Do I look like a vestal virgin to you? How do you think I got this way?" I wondered if this could be a chapter in *The Ten-Second Seduction.*

"Want a T-shirt?"

"I'd prefer one of those toys, if you're giving stuff away."

He laughed. "I'm only allowed to give out shirts. Extra-large is all I have left." When he held it up, I saw the company logo in big bold letters. This was the shirt I would wear during labor. I had no qualms about advertising a sex-toy brand across my pregnancy-heavy boobs.

34 | A Shit Farm in Paradise

Week 39

We hopped into our new-to-us Jeep, stereo included, and headed for our weekly appointment with Dr. Lipstick, since Dr. Enchanté had been called out on an emergency. Chris sat next to me, hands clenched on his lap, endlessly tapping his foot. He still held a grudge against Dr. Lipstick. Her initial dire warning had set the tone for the last five months, and Chris was not ready to forgive her.

Dr. Lipstick's heels clicked on the floor as she entered. Her black, knee-length pencil skirt was cinched at the waist with a thin belt, and a rosy silk blouse completed her outfit. She was shorter than I remembered and her hair was now brown. When she said hello, her lips pursed on the O, and the sheen of her gloss sparkled. Dr. Lipstick extended her hand and I took it. Her handshake was weaker than anticipated, and my firm grip seemed to take her by surprise. I leaned back, put my feet into the stirrups, and spread my legs, ripping away the noisy paper draped across my midsection and throwing it to the floor.

"You're two centimeters dilated," she said after a quick exam.

"What does that mean? Am I having this baby now?"

"It can take weeks for you to fully dilate. Since this is your first child, you will likely carry into October."

"What?"

"Yeah, what?" Chris chimed in.

"After forty-two weeks we'll induce. I'm just preparing you," said the same woman who told me my baby would fall out and die before twenty-four weeks.

I heard my father's voice in my head: "These Sherlocks know shit."

It was obvious she'd had no idea how this pregnancy would go from the beginning, so why had she been so emphatic that I would lose my baby? And why was she casually adding three weeks to my sentence now? It reminded me of the doctor who told my father he was healthy at his checkup two weeks before he died. These physicians were not God, nor were they fortune-tellers. I rested my hand on my belly. This baby would come out on his terms, when he was good and ready, no matter what anybody said or did. That was how it had always been.

"Let's get some manure," Chris said as we left the office.

"What are you talking about?"

"You ever notice how your eyebrows go up to your hairline when you're surprised?"

"Yeah, well, I live my life in a state of disbelief."

"We need manure for the asparagus patch."

"Okay, but let's not go to the same place we tried to buy the door. I think I've been banned from there."

"Yeah, I heard your picture's hanging up in their employee lounge, with darts in it. But that's not where I had in mind."

We stopped at the shop and Chris told me to sit tight while he tended to a customer spewing obscenities because he couldn't get his dead mower off his truck. Using only his brute strength, Chris pulled the machine down. The man offered him a five-dollar tip, but Chris shook his head no and disappeared from my sight line. A few minutes later there was a tug at the Jeep and I grabbed the dashboard as the whole car began rocking back and forth.

"What's going on?" I asked as Chris hopped into the car.

"Hitched the trailer. Let's go."

Chris took me on a joyride through the countryside, taking the sharp turns quicker than I would have liked, especially with a trailer, and driving farther into the hills than I'd ever been. We were surrounded by fields, dotted with crumbling barns and abandoned homes. But it was quiet, and I could just see the first leaves on the trees changing to red.

The Jeep bounced up a rutted driveway flanked by brown dairy cows. "Why don't they build these houses near the road?" I complained as we bumped along.

"Paradise is not built next to a highway," he said as he rolled to a stop. "It must be nice living out here. Quieter."

"Quieter than what? Death? Even the birds don't fly out here."

To the left was a collapsed chicken coop, and behind it a barn that had seen better days. The pitched roof was caved in and only speckles of red suggested that the building once had color. We pulled up to an old double-wide, and two Rottweilers came running out, circling the car.

A wiry older woman with a deep tan that suggested she spent most days outdoors appeared in the doorway. Her hair was tied back and covered with a thin net. "It's okay, they won't kill you," she shouted as she called off Rocco and Peaches.

The midafternoon sun momentarily blinded me when I stepped out of the car. The dogs sniffed me and retreated.

"We need a load of manure. Can you do that for us?" Chris called.

"Sure thing," the woman nodded and then, without another word, headed back into the house for a long time.

In Brooklyn we don't put shit on our vegetables. Intellectually, I knew that this was good for them, that this was how it was done and it was probably better than all the chemicals sprayed on the mass-produced vegetables I grew up eating. But

I was still unnerved by the idea of spreading cow excrement on my food.

The roar of an engine interrupted my thoughts and a big yellow bulldozer made its way through the mud to our shiny Jeep. The woman was at the controls, pulling and pushing them, trying to manage the scooper. I instinctively backed away. She was, after all, hauling a big pile of shit. Then, with no discernible grace, she dumped a load of manure, half onto our trailer and half onto the ground.

"Who's scooping that up?" I asked Chris.

"Try another load?" the woman shouted over the sound of the engine.

Chris gave a thumbs-up.

She disappeared and came back with more manure, this time dumping it directly on the trailer, which sank under the weight.

"Half of one more!" Chris called to her.

"How much manure do we need for our garden?" I said.

"It'll be okay. Gotta spread it on nice and thick. Put your eyebrows down." He reached out and smoothed my forehead.

The woman reappeared with a smaller load, shifted her gears, and began pouring it.

A loud bang caused me to stagger backward. I squatted low to the ground, covering my head with my hands. Looking to see where the gunfire was coming from, I grabbed onto Chris's sleeve, trying to pull him down with me.

"It's the tires." He pulled me back up by the elbow to a standing position and pointed to the trailer, now resting on its rims.

The woman dismounted her dozer and came around to look at our wheels. "Gonna need to tow that," she said, before walking off.

With the sun beating down and the strong smell of manure filling my nostrils, there was no denying that I was stuck on a shit farm in the middle of nowhere with three flat tires.

When she didn't come back, I understood we were not going to be invited into her home to wait for the tow. I found an old tree stump in the shade and, with no small effort, fell back onto it in a seated position. Legs outstretched, I tilted my head hoping to catch a breeze, and looked toward the sky. The weather vane on top of the barn roof turned as the faintest breath of wind wound its way through the treetops. The eaves were brimming with chirping phoebes. There were birds out here after all. The tall grass swayed in the distance, each blade shimmering in the glow of the afternoon sun. Beyond the stench, the chipped paint, and the collapsed roof, there was a quiet beauty out here. Maybe this *was* paradise. I only had to give it a chance.

When I was small, I sat on my father's lap and asked him why he had named me Aileen. "That was your mother's choice," he said. "I wanted to name you Jenny-Sue and move to the country." I watched as a yellow moth landed on a patch of wildflowers and wondered if this was what my dad once had in mind. Maybe he'd pictured himself in a little country cottage, or maybe he would have preferred a great big house with a pool. But he was not a risk taker, and he hadn't even tried to live the life he had dreamed about. He had been paralyzed by doubt and fear. Time and circumstance knocked him down, and he hadn't had the ability to get back up until it was too late. He was delicate and complicated, and he cared so much more than I ever understood until now. He was my best friend, and I wanted him to be my hero. But he wasn't a hero; he was utterly, forgivably human.

After I graduated college, my parents began traveling the world together, falling in love again. Just when my father began truly living for the first time in over twenty years, his life was cut short. So there on that tree stump, I vowed that I would not lose sight of my dreams. I promised my father that no matter what, I would always get back up, just as he had taught me.

Chris called one of his employees to bring tires for the trailer, but the guy showed up with the wrong size. Or they were the right size and he forgot to bring the appropriate tools. Honestly, I'd lost interest in the whole situation. We were going to have to leave the trailer there for now.

We unhitched it from the Jeep and just as we were about to pull away, the woman called out from her doorway, "You gotta pay for that manure."

Chris took out a few bills.

"You're paying her for manure you aren't taking?"

"You want to argue with her?"

She pointed over at me with a long skinny finger. "Sugar pie, you look like you're about to pop, just like them tires." She cackled. "I got three of my own. Honey, it goes so fast." I thought I saw the briefest hint of sadness overcome her as she looked off toward the barn where the phoebes had their nest.

As we pulled away, the faint odor of cow poop lingered on my clothes and in my hair. Somehow, it didn't bother me so much.

35 | Settled, but Not Really

Week 40

My thirty-third birthday had passed quietly, and I was ready to become a mother. But I was far from settled. I would try to focus on a thought, but it would drift away and a new one would replace it. I was fidgety. I kept rearranging my magazines, moving from the couch to the deck and back to the couch. I picked up the phone to call Jackie.

"Are you feeling antsy?" Jackie asked.

"I want to crawl out of my skin."

"You're going into labor. Any day now, I know it."

"The doctor said maybe not for another two weeks!"

"Garbage. Forget the doctor. Listen to me. Right before I went into labor, I ate a tuna fish sandwich. I don't even like tuna. I ate that sandwich and then I went to bed. Next day, bam! Baby baby baby," Jackie said, making me laugh. "Go have sex with your husband, eat some lobster, have a baby. Goodbye."

That evening I most certainly did not eat lobster. I ate nothing. There was no room for food. As for sex, that hadn't happened in five months, but I figured I'd give it a go. To protect the sanctity of my marriage, I will not elaborate on the comedy of errors that ensued, but let's just say Chris finally understood how much weight I had been carrying around all those months. His exact words were: "It felt like I was being rammed in the stomach with a bowling ball." That was really good for my self-esteem.

My eyes shot open at 4:00 a.m. A swirling sensation rushed through my body. I nudged Chris, but he responded with a snoring honk. I tried again, but he wouldn't budge. I considered smothering him with a pillow, but I knew eventually I'd need him to change diapers. Instead, I lay awake for the rest of the night.

In the morning Chris expressed concern when he saw me, eyes wide and unmoving, but I told him it was just my back acting up. I clicked on the television to find Produce Pete talking about apples. Hallelujah. Apple season was upon us.

I passed the day watching the movie *Casanova* and taking baths to ease the pain. When Chris returned at dinnertime, his cell phone was glued to his ear. He was in the middle of one final real estate deal, and I could tell by his tone that it wasn't going well. In between phone conversations he ran out to grab us dinner, and when he came back, he found me lying prone on the floor, trying to ease the tightness and burning in my back. As I breathed through the discomfort, I focused on the ceiling, noticing new Rorschach images that I hadn't seen before . . . a lion, an angel.

Daylight waned over the mountain. The iridescent green hummingbird was alone at the feeder. At 6:00 p.m. I called the after-hours line to check in with my doctor. Dr. Enchanté was unavailable; it was Rosh Hashanah, and he was off for the weekend. The holiday had completely slipped my mind. What kind of Jew had I become, neglecting to acknowledge one of the holiest days of the year? God was, at that moment, jotting down in the Book of Life who would live and who would die, and I had spent the day watching a movie about a gigolo and taking baths. I needed to repent before he doled out retribution, but the good Lord's judgment was too swift for me; the only doctor on call that night was Dr. Lipstick, who was heading home after a double shift.

"You might be in labor," she said.

"I'm not in labor."

"It sounds like you're in labor."

"No. I just have a backache. It comes and goes." I hated this woman. Why was she such an alarmist? First she tells me I'm losing my baby; now she insists I'm in labor. Just calm down, lady. Not everything is a code red.

"Come in. I'm going on forty-eight hours without sleep, but I can wait for you."

Did she just say she hadn't slept in two days? Was she suggesting that there was even a remote possibility that she was going to deliver my baby without having slept for two whole days? It didn't matter. I was not in labor. I told her I'd changed my mind. Everything was fine, really. I would call again in about a week with an update. A sharp pain shot across my lower back. "Don't . . . you . . . think . . . I'd-know-when-I-was-in-labor?" I hissed.

"Most women do," she said.

"Well, this is just a backache."

"Come anyway."

Satchie Red began pawing at my face, circling me in some sort of ancient doggie dance, and slobber began dripping down her jowls right next to my eyeballs. She was barking at me, and when Chris helped me up, she started nipping at my pants, pulling me back.

"What is wrong with everybody?" I lamented as I tried to pet the dog and push her away at the same time.

Chris began herding me to the car. But then his phone rang, and while I waited for him to wrap up his conversation, I ended up on the floor again. Finally, on the third attempt, we made it out the door, but at the last minute he insisted on running back inside to get the hospital bag I had packed.

"We don't need it." I was losing my patience.

"Let's take it just in case." He threw it in the trunk.

I tried to climb into the front seat, but I couldn't sit up, so Chris hoisted me into the back.

Every few minutes on the way to the hospital, the pain began to pulse and I'd shout obscenities. As we crossed over the Kingston-Rhinecliff Bridge, Chris broke his silence. "Aileen, you're screaming in five-minute intervals. I've been timing you. I don't want to offend you. Don't be mad at me, okay? Promise you will not be mad when I say this."

"What could you possibly say to make me mad right now?"

"I think maybe you're in labor."

I gripped a rawhide dog bone that had been left on the seat, about to throw it at his head, but I hesitated. Perhaps he was right. If so, this was the moment I had been waiting for since I was four years old.

36 | The Fibroids Ate My Baby

Go Time

Anne, my doula, met us in the hospital parking lot and asked me to take a deep breath and ground myself to the earth beneath my feet. I pushed her aside. There was no time to breathe; I needed to see a doctor. Within minutes a nurse's hands were up my lady parts, trying to determine how dilated I was. She confirmed what everybody except me had already known. I was in labor.

Once settled into the hospital room, Chris ran out to make phone calls while Anne rubbed my feet. I inhaled through the pain, focusing on the little dots in the panels of the drop ceiling. Anne dimmed the lights and turned on the chanting music I had brought. Here I was, listening to Krishna Das on Rosh Hashanah. I wondered what Rachel would think. I wanted to call her, tell her it was time, see if she had any last-minute advice, tell her to pray for me.

I lost myself in a song about living in the presence of the Lord. The Jewish religion says there is only one God, but it didn't matter to me where this spiritual presence came from, as long as it was inside me. I wanted to tell this to Rachel. I wanted her to know, it's what is in your heart, it's how your soul connects to another soul, it's through your acts of kindness. Your acts of love. That is how you live in the presence of the Lord.

Dr. Lipstick strolled into the room and turned up the lights with zero regard for the fact that she was interrupting my epiphany. The first thing I noticed were her bare lips.

272

What, no Chanel today? I guess we're in the trenches now, lady. Then, because the nurse's report of my dilated cervix wasn't enough, she, too, manhandled me.

When she left, my eyes welled up. I had made it to forty weeks, which would have been such a great reason to cry, but that had nothing to do with it. "I miss Satchie Red," I wailed, searching for a tissue.

That damn dog, who was fickle and hated to be touched, who was too evolved for her owners, had become, in the last five months, my saving grace. And the thing is, I knew that once this baby arrived, that dog's life was going to be a world of suck.

Then I pulled my shit together. I spent the rest of that long night breathing. No drugs: just me, Krishna Das, and my doula. Chris was vaguely there, too, but shortly after we arrived, he fell into a deep sleep in the designated support-person chair. A meteorite could have landed on the steps of the birthing center, and the man would not have stirred.

When Dr. Lipstick came in to check my cervix again, I screamed bloody murder, trying to twist myself away, wondering why every single person who gave me advice all these months failed to mention that multiple people would be checking to see how dilated I was, and when they did, it would take every ounce of willpower not to kick them in the face. It was open season on my vagina. The nurse apologized for the doctor when she was done, but it felt more perfunctory than genuine. Chris continued to snore with abandon. He was on my hit list, too.

As the night wore on, I began to entertain the idea of an epidural. I had fought the good fight. I had been in labor for twenty-two hours and the end was nowhere in sight. The anesthesiologist gave me an intrathecal, which would temporarily numb my midsection, giving me a reprieve, but still allow me to push when the time came. It wore off in forty minutes. I asked for another dose, but he had gone home for the night and the nurse insisted it was too soon for more drugs. I continued with the deep breathing, hoping the tide would turn and this baby would make an appearance. Two hours later, when I could no longer tolerate the pain, the nurse paged the anesthesiologist. When he still hadn't shown up after another hour, Anne suggested the birthing tub.

As the water filled around me, my muscles relaxed and I hoisted myself into a squatting position. I looked at the clock. It was 6:00 a.m. I decreed that this baby had until 8:00 a.m. to come into this world. After that, I was packing it in. We could try again in a year or two. "You hear me, little man? Eight o'clock. Say farewell to the Monsters. They are not your siblings. You have no attachment to them. You need to come out." I actually said this to the baby inside my body, as if he were going to wrap up his PowerPoint presentation, take final questions, and exit my uterus in a suit and tie.

There was a commotion in the hallway and Chris's frantic voice: "Where's my wife? Have you seen my wife?" The man had finally risen from his gentle slumber.

When Chris saw me, he stopped in his tracks. "Wow." He stood in the corner of the room. "You look beautiful," he whispered. It felt like the first time he had seen me in months.

The edges of my lips turned up. "I do?"

"Yeah, you do." He sat down on the side of the tub.

I could have stayed there for hours. There was no pain in that tub. I was strong and powerful. I was rising up from a dark place, naked and reborn without Kate Spade purses and couture dresses. Stripped down, with this hard, round belly, I was sure of who I was and where I wanted to be.

Unfortunately, I had to pee. Two hours later my bladder was so full that the nurse insisted I come out of the tub. It was the first time in my life that I'd been able to hold it, but after another fifteen minutes she cited some medical reason as to why it was bad for the baby and pulled the plug on the drain.

At 8:30 a.m., almost four hours after he was first paged, the anesthesiologist strolled into my room with a smile on his face, looking well rested. *I hope you didn't rush. I wouldn't want my twenty-eight hours of contractions to have interrupted your morning latte.* Darts flew out of my eyes and wiped that grin right off his face. I looked around for Chris, but he was gone.

The anesthesiologist held up the needle. "Wait! Don't! I need Chris!"

"Someone find her husband," Nurse Kim, the morning nurse, said. She was a short, stern woman with a head full of curly gray hair pulled back in a ponytail.

They finally found him on his phone in the parking lot.

"Where were you? The anesthesiologist is here."

"Sorry, I had to call one of the neighbors to let out Satchie Red."

"My Satchie Red." I started crying again. "She's all alone. I need my dog, RIGHT NOW!" Who were these evil people that didn't allow dogs in birthing centers?

"Hold on. Hold on. Don't move," I heard the anesthesiologist say as he prepped my back for the second intrathecal right in the middle of a contraction. Chris stood in front of me squeezing my hands for support. I lifted my gaze to meet his just in time to see his eyes roll to the back of his head. He stumbled right into Anne. "Grab him! Grab him! Get him a chair," Anne called out to hospital personnel swarming the room. All attention was on Chris, who managed not to hit the floor, instead landing in a chair that a nurse had pushed under him. "Breathe, Chris, breathe. It's going to be all right. You're doing great," said Anne.

First we meet in a grocery store, then he passes out during labor. Were our whole lives destined to be one cliché after another?

When the second injection wore off forty minutes later, the anesthesiologist came back and gave me something stronger.

After that I began to lose what little cool I had left. I needed alone time.

"Everybody out, right now. Everybody."

Miraculously, they listened to me, each one filing out the door.

I felt an animalistic shift. I closed my eyes. I was in the woods, giving birth like a she-wolf to her cubs under a canopy of crisp green leaves. When I opened my eyes, I could no longer feel anything from my waist down. My contractions slowed, and Dr. Lipstick came back, pushing Pitocin to move things along. I acquiesced, but it didn't work. I spiked a fever. Somewhere I had an infection, and my baby's heart rate was skyrocketing. This was emergency territory.

Dr. Lipstick approached cautiously, sizing me up to see if I would gnash my teeth, but I let her have her way with me without protest. I couldn't feel a thing; she could have driven a Mack truck through my vagina and it wouldn't have fazed me.

"You're nine centimeters dilated and ten is the lucky number. I can push that last bit open, but I'm going to suggest a C-section. The baby is jammed up against your pelvic bone."

"I can push."

"You're too exhausted to push. Besides, you have no feeling in your lower body. We'd have to wait for the epidural to wear off, and the baby's heart rate is worrisome."

"I can push right now. Let me push." I couldn't push. There was no way in hell I could push. If I tried, it would have to be some sort of Vulcan mind trick.

It was 11:00 a.m. and I needed an emergency C-section, but it was still Rosh Hashanah and a Sunday. These Jewish holidays go on forever. Apparently they needed two doctors to perform the surgery. Dr. Enchanté was in synagogue, and there were no other OB-GYNs on call. It took some negotiating, but a doctor from another practice finally agreed to assist.

I turned to Nurse Kim. "I need to wait for my family to arrive before going in. Chris called them, but I don't know when they'll get here."

"Your in-laws have been here for two hours."

"No one mentioned this?"

"They didn't want to bother you." Nurse Kim shrugged.

"When my family comes, please send my brother in first. I need to talk to him." The person I really needed now was my father, but I hoped my brother could step up to the task.

"How will I know it's them?" said Nurse Kim.

"Believe me. You'll know."

Not long after, there was a ruckus outside my window. People were yelling in the parking lot. I heard a buzzer, and my brother's voice shouted into the intercom, "We're here for Aileen Weintraub."

"I don't think that's her name anymore!" My mother yelled, pressing the intercom again, this time saying Chris's last name. "I think she changed her name," my sister-in-law chimed in.

These people didn't even know my name, and here I was contributing to their gene pool. The energy of the birthing center moved toward chaos. The Brooklyn Jews were in the house.

Mark stepped into my room alone. "Hi there."

"They want to cut me open."

"So what? *I* won't feel a thing."

"That's the best you can do? What would Dad say?"

"I'm pretty sure that's what Dad would say. Seriously, he would say, 'Look what you've been through the last five months. This is cake.' Then he'd go have a cigarette and yell at Mom."

And that's when my mother, who had been waiting outside the door and could no longer control herself, came running in. "*Mamaleh!* How are you doing, my *shayna maidel?* What do you need? You're going to be fine."

My brother turned to her. "Mom, deep breaths. You're going to be fine, too."

The in-laws followed. They all began mingling, talking over one another and forgetting I was there. "It would be nice if you could make an appearance now," I murmured. But my father hated hospitals.

And then a whisper. "Whataya worried about? You'll be fine. It's already been taken care of." Both my parents had promised I'd be fine, so maybe it was true.

The operating room was sterile and bare, a far cry from the cozy oasis I had created down the hall. "This time I'm giving you a combination I've never tried on anyone else," said the anesthesiologist. I waited for him to laugh, but he was dead serious. He explained that since I'd already had a lot of drugs, he'd have to make sure there were no unusual interactions. In other circumstances I would have insisted on a clearer explanation, but I was focusing my fight elsewhere. The nurses, different ones now, put up a huge white sheet across my chest so I couldn't see what was going on below. Feeling too weak and too tired to talk, I asked Anne and Chris to make conversation to distract me. Five months in bed and I was starting out motherhood with a sleep deficit. There was pulling and tugging, but no pain. Dr. Lipstick said something, but I didn't catch it. Then the head of a blue wrinkled creature popped over the sheet.

I flinched.

Oh my God! The fibroids ate my baby! What the hell is that?

There was a huge dent in my child's head.

As if reading my thoughts, Dr. Lipstick said, "The impression will go away. Your baby is healthy." I turned to see Chris and the nurses hovering around this tiny human. Using the back of his pointer finger, Chris tentatively stroked the baby's leg, awestruck. Hormones, drugs, and emotions surged together, meeting at an apex of satisfaction and desire. Right then, gutted open like a fish, I fell in love with my son's father all over again.

The nurse swaddled my wailing newborn and brought him over to me. But I wasn't ready; I couldn't touch him. Here, with my insides exposed on the table, our first meeting, I was afraid I wouldn't be good enough. Anne placed him next to my face so I could see his soft, now pink, baby body, and when I said, "Hello there," he stopped crying. He knew me, he knew my voice, and right then, arms tied down, bright lights shining in my eyes, among the beeps and drips and official doctor jargon, I had become a mother.

37 | After Birth

Post-delivery Blur

The baby was outside my body. But the Monsters were still there.

"Anne, come take a look." Dr. Lipstick pulled my doula over to the other side of the curtain. "Those are her fibroids," she continued.

"Wow." Anne nodded, trying to maintain her professionalism.

The doctor turned to the room at large and asked if anyone else wanted to see, as if I were an exhibit at the Coney Island Freak Show. Five dollars a pop to see the lady with the Monster Fibroids, come one, come all.

"Can you take them out?" I managed from behind the sheet.

"No, you'll hemorrhage. That's for another day," Dr. Lipstick replied. I felt a lot of shmooshing and heard the glopping of bodily fluids. I was getting restless. Anne was talking to me about the baby, but it was difficult to respond. My mouth was sandpaper and the people on the other side of the sheet were fondling my insides. I needed this to be over.

"How much longer?" I said.

"She's slurring her words," Anne called to the anesthesiologist.

"Not slurring," I said.

"You're slurring."

"No."

"A little bit."

Turns out, when you're slurring your words, you have no idea that you're slurring. Funny how that works.

"It's fine, just the medication," I heard the unattached voice of the anesthesiologist. He adjusted one of the many tubes dangling off my body.

I was wheeled back into what kind of looked like the same room but was definitely not the same room. Or maybe it was. Something was different. The doctors were tilted and the light left a fuzzy afterglow on the tissue box and medical receptacles. It felt a little déjà vu–y.

A bunch of medical people I hadn't seen before surrounded my bed. I asked for water. When there was no acknowledgment, I wondered if they could hear me. Everything felt far away. "Hello? I can see the bottle right there. Can you hand it to me?"

A nurse laughed. "It'll wear off soon," she said, flipping her hand absentmindedly.

Was I doing something funny? Were my words not coming out of my mouth the way I was hearing them? Maybe I was still slurring. In my head I said, *Really, bitch? You're laughing at me because I need water?* But on the outside, I just felt confused. Something wasn't translating. All I knew for certain was that my throat was raw and dry; it felt like it was on fire.

"Anne. Where's my doula?" I asked, glad to remember I had an advocate. When she heard me calling her, she appeared. With the nurse's permission, Anne handed me a water bottle.

I fumbled around, but my hands weren't grasping correctly. Anne took the bottle back and opened it for me. I took a small sip. And then . . . I stopped breathing. There was no air. I grabbed at my chest, eyes bulging. The anesthesiologist rushed toward me, throwing me over the bed railing. Someone else was pounding on my back. Another technician grabbed my arms and raised them over my head. All I could think was, *It's a good thing I can't feel any of this.*

Nobody was laughing now.

I drew in a delicious gasp of air. Well that sobered me right up. The room was crystal clear. Dr. Lipstick came in just as the commotion was dying down.

"I nearly killed your patient," the anesthesiologist quipped. "Must have been the cocktail of medications." Dr. Lipstick chuckled. I failed to find the humor in any of this.

Chris came in and knelt beside the bed.

"I made it through five months of bed rest and then nearly died from a sip of water."

"Well, you're okay now."

"That's the way I roll."

Nurse Kim was behind him, holding our baby. She placed my child in my arms. He was wearing a purple knit hat. Our heartbeats synced. I touched the tip of his tiny nose to make sure he was real.

Our families filed in to welcome our new joy and hear the baby's name, which we had kept secret. In the Jewish tradition, you take the first letter of the name of someone who has died, so we told them we were using an R for my father, Richard. But they had to guess from there.

They threw out a few names but hadn't even come close.

A few more tries and Chris offered some hints. "It's the name of a gun, a razor, and an eighties television show."

"Remington!" my sister-in-law finally guessed.

Chris and I simultaneously turned to gauge his mother's reaction, knowing that she wouldn't approve of the nontraditional name. One side of her mouth was raised and her head had jolted back, eyebrows scrunched together.

"And the middle name . . ." I began, still looking at Nadine.

"Is my father's name," Chris finished the sentence. My mother-in-law let out a gasp and began falling backward but then grabbed the bed railing and got a hold of herself. There was no love lost between her and her first husband.

With the official announcement of our child's name, the paparazzi swarmed, blinding me and the baby with their flashes.

"This is all lovely," I said, shielding my eyes and cradling our son to my chest, "but I just went through thirty-six hours of torture. You need to stop flashing lights at me." They couldn't help themselves. They had all been on this journey with me, and now we were together and safe and the baby was finally here. But when Nurse Kim saw me trying to roll away and block the baby's eyes from the lights, she kicked everyone out.

Nurse Kim and I formed a bond I never would have expected possible from someone I had just met. She helped me in ways that no other human being ever had, except my own mother. While I recovered at the hospital, she bathed me, took me to the bathroom, and dressed me when I could barely move. She even stuck one of those giant maxi pads between my legs when I got out of the shower. I was humbled by her. She was gentle and patient while I tried to breastfeed, and when the doctors were concerned because I had a headache that wouldn't quit for three days, she reassured me.

On our last full day at the hospital, the anesthesiologist paid me a visit. They couldn't release me until they figured out the cause of the headache. He was going to do a test to determine whether or not I had a spinal leak. I didn't know if I could handle any more probing.

He opened the blinds. "Look out the window."

I turned my head, focusing on the freshly mown grass outside.

"All good. If you had a leak, you wouldn't be able to stand the bright light."

"That was your scientific test? Look out the window? How much do you get paid an hour?"

"Quite a lot, actually." He raised his eyebrows and left the room.

As soon as my mother heard that I wasn't in need of surgery or further testing, she barged in with an agenda. "We need to talk about the bris. Everything's *fakakt*. I have a list of about fifty people. It's going to be the day of Yom Kippur eve. Your brother doesn't want to wait on line to pick up the appetizing because the bagel store will be too crowded with holiday orders. What do you want to do?" The source of my headache was becoming clear.

She sat down cross-legged on the floor next to the bed and spread out her papers: lists, menus, and names of *mohels* to do the circumcision. Then she ticked off the guests she'd be inviting. This was all for her. I'd agreed to this out of some moral obligation, and now my brother wouldn't pick up the platters she'd ordered in Brooklyn. There was no other place to order kosher food on such short notice before the holiday. I couldn't have fifty Brooklyn Jews travel upstate and not hand them a decent bagel.

"If he can't be bothered picking up the food, Ma, that's fine. He doesn't have to come. I'll let him know."

"What? What do you mean he doesn't have to come?"

"I have mixed feelings about this anyway. If it's going to be difficult, we don't need a bris."

"Over my dead body! My grandson needs a bris," she said.

"Cancel the bris," I said, matching her tone.

With all the painkillers coursing through my body, I can't pretend to remember what happened after that, but it culminated in my calling the nurse and my mother storming out, while my mother-in-law looked on in horror at the spectacle.

Nurse Kim told me I could go home the next day; all I had to do was sign a paper that said I was ready to be discharged. Umm, no. I told her I just needed a few more weeks. These people were taking good care of me, serving what turned out to be decent food, helping me with the baby, and their television had more cable channels than mine did. All I had to do was press a button and someone would come and do whatever I asked. Why would I leave? And what about the baby? What the hell was I supposed to do with him? I had no idea how to take care of one of these things. Dressing my Holly Hobby doll, years of babysitting experience, useless.

Alas, the next morning Chris pulled around with the Jeep, and we posed for a farewell picture on the steps of the birthing center. My mother had knit a white coming-home sweater-and-pants set for the baby. Getting it on his body was like trying to dress an octopus. These tiny little creatures were a lot more trouble than they looked and completely offended by clothing.

Chris held up the car seat and we both wondered, *What in God's good name is supposed to happen here?* We'd assumed one of the nurses would know how it worked, but turns out that wasn't part of their job description. By the time we figured it out, our baby was thoroughly disgusted with us, and his wailing was scaring the other pregnant women. We settled him into the car, where Nadine was waiting in the backseat. He wrapped his little hand around her finger, holding her tight the whole way home.

The leaves were turning, specks of yellow and red mingled with green. I could smell the pine trees as we pulled into our driveway. Chris helped me out of the car and I sat on the bench in our yard. He brought Remington over, placing him beside me in his car seat. Satchie Red came barreling toward me, barking and whining, then sat on her haunches demanding an explanation for my long absence.

"We gave her the baby's onesie yesterday to prepare her, but she tossed it right out of her bed," Nadine said.

I took Remington out of the car seat and brought him to Satchie Red's level. "Satchie Red, meet your new baby." She turned her head away, unimpressed.

"Come in, I have lunch ready," my mother said from the doorway. The fight about the bris had been resolved. My mother called the bagel store and strongly encouraged the owner to allow my brother to bypass the long line for pickup.

I sat on the bench with Remington in my arms, looking up at the house: my former prison. It was just a house, and not a bad one at that. Despite my fear that it would collapse at the exact moment this child entered the world, it was still standing. For five months I thought everything was falling down around me, but here we were, stronger than ever.

I had been freed from my confinement, and now I was finding it hard to reenter the house. It would be different now, I reminded myself. I could come and go at will. I had a beautiful baby. It had all worked out. But I knew it wouldn't be easy to move on. There had been no mention of bed rest since the birth, but it wasn't something I would soon forget. I would walk that path of healing, privately and invisibly, for years, just as my father had.

I would never really know what caused his years of depression or if he ever came to terms with the demons that haunted him. I regretted that I couldn't help him more or understand him better when he was alive, but I could continue to learn from him. With any luck, I would have the same camaraderie with my child that my father and I shared toward the end of his life. If nothing else, I'd teach my son to stand up for himself and not care what anyone else thought as long as he was doing what felt right. And I'd let him make mistakes, no matter how hard it might be for both of us, so he, too, could find his own way.

"Aileen, are you with us?" My mother was standing in front of me, pulling me by the arm. "Come already. I have egg salad."

What could be bad when you have egg salad? I didn't even have to eat it off a tray table anymore. I made my way up the stairs and into the kitchen, and we sat down together at the table, Remington content on my lap.

"You're a pro already," my mother said.

Satchie Red came over and stood next to me. Now that the baby was inside the house, he was worthy of investigation. Satchie Red yawned and let out a great big moan. The baby lolled his little blond head, trying to focus on the animal sniffing his toes. The dog raised her nose up, inhaling the baby's scent. Then she went over to the onesie that she had previously cast aside. She sniffed it and came back. She sniffed the baby one more time and looked up at him. She knew this person was here to stay. Just then Remington made a tiny little squeak and baby puke gushed out of his mouth—right onto Satchie Red's head. Satchie Red skittered away, sliding in the fluid. She shook her whole body and then retreated to her bed, tail between her legs, where she licked white curds off her paws, thoroughly disgusted.

"Well, looks like my milk came in," I said, taking a bite of my egg salad sandwich.

38 | Mother

Week 1

I had been home for two days and had graduated from baby incubator to milk dispenser. I settled the baby in his pack 'n' play, and then I collapsed on the sofa. Just when I thought I might catch a moment's rest, the dog came running at me full force, jumped up, and grabbed a boob in her mouth. I pushed her away and she nipped at my shirt again. I loved my dog. I didn't want to become one of those women who neglected her animal when the baby arrived, but I had to draw a line. I was not going to breastfeed a canine. Satchie Red, who had always mostly ignored me, now, for the first time in her life, wanted attention. There would be no rest. Instead, I got up to eat while I had the chance, making sure I had enough sustenance to provide for my baby vulture's next ravenous feeding.

When he began to wail, I picked him up and brought him to the Papasan chair in the nursery, where I sat cross-legged, stuffing my giant raw nipple into his mouth. Chris had somehow completed the renovations while I was in the hospital. I have no idea if he hired a crew or if he did it himself in between hospital visits and work, or if it was divine intervention, but I wasn't going to question it.

The house felt fresh and crisp. As far as I could tell, nothing was in imminent danger of falling down anymore. We even had a door! It was as though at the exact moment my son was ripped from my womb, some sort of equilibrium within the universe had balanced everything out. The baby had been sucking the life force out of me, Chris, *and* the house, but now our child was here and all was calm.

I looked down at the faint dent on my son's forehead, running my finger over it. It would be gone soon. He had been pressed up against the Monsters for so long that his neck muscles had strengthened, and he could already hold up his head on his own. He had the bluest eyes and wisps of blond hair on the tippy top of his head, and was the spitting image of the baby in the photograph on his dresser dated 1933, the year my father was born.

When we were done nursing, I gathered him close and began the slow, painful process of coming to a standing position. My foot caught in the chair and I lurched forward, baby in arms. There was no stopping the momentum. Cupping his head with my hands to break the blow, I slammed my knee down hard on the wood floor. Two gigantic milk-filled breasts bounced on top of him, smooshing his face. There was a thud and then we were both still. I lifted my body, preparing for the worst. Six days old—had I killed him already? I looked at him. I could swear the kid raised one eyebrow as if to say, "What the fuck, lady?" But he wasn't crying—not until he saw my face, which was twisted in horror. It dawned on me that this human being was depending on me for guidance. My reaction dictated his. This was parenthood. I met his big blue eyes. "Don't worry, kid, I've got this. We're going to be okay."

With fifty people set to come to my house the next day to have a party for my baby's penis, I asked Chris to meet me for lunch at a café. I was free from my shackles, and even though it took almost an hour to pack the diaper bag and dress the baby, I was emotionally rejuvenated. I took tiny, excruciating steps, every unplanned movement, sneeze, and twitch feeling like it would tear my healing scar open. Recovery was slow, because of both the surgery and the months of bed rest that preceded it, but I was allowed out of the house for as long as I wanted.

Chris and I sat at an outdoor table at the café, Remington sleeping beside me in his stroller. With the gestational diabetes gone, I ordered all varieties of carbs: panini, chips, sweetened iced tea. Local folks I hadn't seen in months, who had no knowledge of my ordeal, peered into the carriage to get a glimpse of the baby. That fall day, sitting in an outdoor café with my little family was everything I had ever wanted.

The Brooklyn Jews arrived in waves, filling the house with coats, gifts, and boxes of rugelach. With every new arrival, the house bulged with *kinehoras* and *mazels* until Chris wondered out loud if the family room could support the weight. The women went to work in the kitchen, unwrapping, plating, stirring, and cooking, their long skirts swooshing as they chopped, sliced, and set the silver. Husbands milled around on the deck admiring the view, asking Chris questions about our expansive yard, our garden, and the integrity of the barn. For the most part I stayed in the nursery, listening from afar and signing official documents the *mohel* produced. But eventually I couldn't resist venturing out. The hum of the house was protective and welcoming. My father's cousins, neighbors from down the road, my friends from the 'hood all showed up, including Watson, who stood on the steps and declared, "It's not that bad up here." I gave both him and his wife long hugs as their kids scampered in.

Chris's mother was surprised to see so many people squeezed into our old farmhouse. She stood just out of the way in the hall, wanting to help but not quite sure how to enter the cyclone of activity. I understood her hesitation. It was like to trying to jump onto a moving Tilt-A-Whirl, only with knives and herring flying around.

When the time came, my brother called for me, and I carried the baby across the worn brown carpet into the living room, surrounded by friends and family. No one seemed to notice or care that the room was stuck in a seventies time warp. One by one, I looked around at each of their faces as they chatted, gesticulated, and threw back glasses of celebratory wine. My two worlds had finally collided in this space overlooking the Shawangunk Ridge; Brooklyn had come to me. There was laughter and love in that room.

Everyone quieted down as I handed the baby to the *mohel.* I moved toward the back because I was told it's too much for a mother to bear, but in the end, my baby, the taste of sweet wine on his tongue and not a little bit of numbing lotion on his nether region, did not make a peep. It was over in a jiffy, and he was back in my arms. I showed him off to the crowd as my mother's friends formed a protective circle around me, not consciously, but because each one of them considered me her own.

Now it was a full-blown party, and joy permeated every rickety corner. My brother was introducing himself to anyone he didn't already know, trying to find out their political affiliations. Mud-soaked children ran up and down the driveway, as my mother pushed lox and sable like a meth dealer. "You want a little? You're doing me a favor. Take it." As I watched the festivities, I noticed that Jackie was missing. I had a feeling that, like an angel who came into my life just when I needed her, I would be hearing from her a lot less.

By the time everyone was ready to leave, I was exhausted and my pain medication was wearing off, but I rallied to express my gratitude and say goodbye. With fifty guests, we had gotten creative with the parking, and many had lined up their cars in the field across the street. Watson was the first to reappear speckled with mud after saying his goodbyes.

"Minivan's stuck. I have to get out of here. It's going to be dark soon."

"Watson, it's 3:30 in the afternoon."

"Don't be nitpicky. There are no streetlights here. We need to get out. We need to get out now."

"Okay. Let's not panic."

"We may have to sleep over. Do you have space for us to sleep over? It's Erev Yom Kippur, you know."

As I was heading toward the door, my brother appeared. "My minivan is stuck. I'm spinning my wheels."

Soon others came back making the same declaration. It was amusing at first, but the lightheartedness faded as the sun dipped below the mountains.

Chris brought out metal grates for traction, country folk took the wheel, and everybody pushed. Mud splattered, grass flew, tires roared, and engines whirred. The men took turns rocking the cars back and forth, to no avail.

"Get the diesel," I called to Chris.

"Big city editor has a diesel, you believe that shit?" my brother Mark quipped to Watson.

Chris came back with the diesel, blocked the road, and hitched chains to one minivan at a time. My father's cousin, a feisty older woman draped in cashmere and silk, took the wheel of one of the cars. "Keep it straight, keep it straight," she was advised, and to this day she swears she did, but I have a photo saying otherwise. People began arguing strategy. My brother took over his own steering wheel as four other men pushed. "Go, go, go," they shouted, but just as we thought his car was free, Mark slammed his brakes, afraid to pull out onto the road. "In the city we don't floor it without looking." His wheels began to spin again, and we had to start over.

One by one the cars were pulled free and sent on their way. I stood and witnessed it all, in no condition to be useful other than to provide moral support peppered with the occasional sarcastic commentary. With the last car on solid ground, Chris came to my side and put his arm around me as we watched my closest friends and family depart. It was hard to see them go, especially Watson, who had promised to come up and visit again sometime. "I could see it happening," he said, giving me a final hug goodbye.

My husband pulled me close, my face pressing against his mud-covered shirt. I laughed and tried to struggle free, but he held me tight in his grip. We had a long way to go to heal our relationship, especially with the stress of a new baby, but I had faith we would persevere.

Watson honked his horn as he pulled away. I thought of *The Ten-Second Seduction.* Covered in mud, hitched to a man who sells power equipment, with a post-pregnancy body to boot, I was no longer a contender to be *the* seductress of Ulster County. It didn't matter. There was a whole new life unfolding before me. The past was behind me. It was a past filled with beauty and pain, and not a small dose of uncertainty. It was a past brimming with the delicious memories of my father, and though I wanted to hold on, I knew I had to let go if I was going to create a worthwhile future.

The last red streaks of daylight were fading behind the mountain. My father was there, watching all of this, laughing. I heard his voice crystal clear: "You see, Kabeen, I told you, it's all been taken care of."

I studied the curve of Chris's cheekbones. His face had a new hardness to it. He was strong and solid. As though he were part of the conversation with my father, he said, "Things always have a way of working out."

I reached up to kiss him on the cheek, but he turned and met my lips. Then he headed toward the diesel while I returned to the house to find my son. My mother-in-law was cuddling Remington, sitting and chatting with the last few guests in the family room. Standing before her, she placed him in my waiting arms. I cradled him to my body and carried him to his room, where we sat nursing on the Papasan. Through the closed door, I could hear the sweet din of laughter.

Acknowledgments

One of the best things a writer can do while writing a memoir is to surround herself with people who believe in her more than she believes in herself. I am so lucky that the following people have cajoled, offered tough love, read, reread, read some more, edited, proofread, held my hand, and could see something in my work that I had yet to see myself.

First and foremost, to my agent Susan Cohen for her kindness, dedication, and thoughtful advice—thank you for all that you do. I am so grateful to my amazing editor Courtney Ochsner, along with Sara Springsteen, Rosemary Sekora, Debbie Anderson, Tayler Lord, Laura Buis, and the rest of the UNP team. This book wouldn't have been possible without you.

The seeds for *Knocked Down* were planted when I organized a book club for overworked, stressed-out moms who were hoping to read something other than *Goodnight Moon* for the hundredth time. We chose *The Happiness Project* by Gretchen Rubin. Inspired by that book, I called my dear friend Kerrie Baldwin and told her my idea. She encouraged me to go for it.

I began writing whenever I had a free moment—the grocery store line, waiting in my car at school pickup, in doctors' offices and cafés. When I had thirty pages, I read an excerpt to my brother, and he said, "I think you have something here." I showed chapters to Liza Darnton, talking structure and arcs while our kids played in the sandbox.

When I began the arduous process of submitting, writing through rejection and disappointment, Ed Serken said, "Shut

out the noise. Write your story and keep going until it's done."
He had no idea what he was getting himself into because he
has been reading pages ever since.

Finally I had a draft. I didn't know what to do with it so I tied
it up in a plastic bag and threw it in the back of my closet. Days
later, Erica Chase Salerno invited me to a writing group. This
group was a "total game changer," as Erica liked to say. And
so JADE was formed, an acronym for our initials that included
Jennifer Wulfe and Donna Eis. We met every other Monday
for two years in a coffee shop that served the best red velvet
cupcakes with chocolate filling, and it was there that Erica
encouraged me to dig deeper, be raw, and get real. She did
this mostly by shouting enthusiastically and putting red check
marks on my pages. Then we spread out the manuscript on
Donna's giant table and weaved in themes and threads and
ate a lot of cheese. Okay, mostly I ate the cheese. Shortly after,
Erica passed away, and I didn't know whom else I could trust
to tell me the hard truths.

That's when Blair Glaser stepped into my life, read my book,
and so generously invited me to a self-made writers' retreat
where I spent five days cutting my precious darlings.

Sara Munson tells me beautiful things about my writing that
I want to frame and hang on the wall because she knows I live
in the land of anxiety. Risë Finkle, Heidi Garnett, and Wanda
Sherman have been there through the ups and downs, mostly
with delicious food that feeds my heart and soul.

Thank you to the SUNY Ulster crew, who are incredible writ-
ers and educators and say things like, "You got this girl," and,
"Trust the process." To Greg Payan, my dear friend and out-
standing photographer, along with Kathleen Elliot. To Stacey
Arenella and Susan Forster, who read the final draft. To the
Binders. To Katharine Daugherty, who generously provided
me space to write at Drop Forge and Toole. To my high school
English teacher Gail Katz, who sparked my love of writing

when she assigned *The Grapes of Wrath* and was the first person to believe in my work. To my childhood librarian at the Kings Highway Branch whose name I wish I could remember and who made RIF so much fun. To Mandy Patinkin, Kathryn Grody, Sue William Silverman, Sari Botton, Nava Atlas, Aspen Matis, Cameron Dezen Hammon, and Elissa Altman—I am so grateful for your kind, supportive words, which gave me the confidence to release this book into the world.

And finally, most important, to my mother and father. To my husband, Christopher, the guardian of my solitude and without whom not one word of this story would have been written. And to my strong, athletic, brilliant son, Remington, you are my everything.

In the American Lives Series

Hannah and the Mountain: Notes toward a Wilderness Fatherhood
by Jonathan Johnson

Local Wonders: Seasons in the Bohemian Alps
by Ted Kooser

A Certain Loneliness: A Memoir
by Sandra Gail Lambert

Bigger than Life: A Murder, a Memoir
by Dinah Lenney

What Becomes You
by Aaron Raz Link
and Hilda Raz

Queen of the Fall: A Memoir of Girls and Goddesses
by Sonja Livingston

The Virgin of Prince Street: Expeditions into Devotion
by Sonja Livingston

Anything Will Be Easy after This: A Western Identity Crisis
by Bethany Maile

Such a Life
by Lee Martin

Turning Bones
by Lee Martin

In Rooms of Memory: Essays
by Hilary Masters

Island in the City: A Memoir
by Micah McCrary

Between Panic and Desire
by Dinty W. Moore

To Hell with It: Of Sin and Sex, Chicken Wings, and Dante's Entirely Ridiculous, Needlessly Guilt-Inducing "Inferno"
by Dinty W. Moore

Let Me Count the Ways: A Memoir
by Tomás Q. Morín

Shadow Migration: Mapping a Life
by Suzanne Ohlmann

Meander Belt: Family, Loss, and Coming of Age in the Working-Class South
by M. Randal O'Wain

Sleep in Me
by Jon Pineda

The Solace of Stones: Finding a Way through Wilderness
by Julie Riddle

Works Cited: An Alphabetical Odyssey of Mayhem and Misbehavior
by Brandon R. Schrand

Thoughts from a Queen-Sized Bed
by Mimi Schwartz

My Ruby Slippers: The Road Back to Kansas
by Tracy Seeley

The Fortune Teller's Kiss
by Brenda Serotte

Gang of One: Memoirs of a Red Guard
by Fan Shen

Just Breathe Normally
by Peggy Shumaker

How to Survive Death and Other Inconveniences
by Sue William Silverman

The Pat Boone Fan Club: My Life as a White Anglo-Saxon Jew
by Sue William Silverman

Scraping By in the Big Eighties
by Natalia Rachel Singer

Sky Songs: Meditations on Loving a Broken World
by Jennifer Sinor

In the Shadow of Memory
by Floyd Skloot

Secret Frequencies: A New York Education
by John Skoyles

The Days Are Gods
by Liz Stephens

Phantom Limb
by Janet Sternburg

This Jade World
by Ira Sukrungruang

When We Were Ghouls: A Memoir of Ghost Stories
by Amy E. Wallen

Knocked Down: A High-Risk Memoir
by Aileen Weintraub

Yellowstone Autumn: A Season of Discovery in a Wondrous Land
by W. D. Wetherell

This Fish Is Fowl: Essays of Being
by Xu Xi

To order or obtain more information on these or other University of Nebraska Press titles, visit nebraskapress.unl.edu.